"Dr Eden does parents of young children a great service in *Obesity Prevention for Children*. He provides a lucid and succinct review of the causes of early childhood obesity, along with many straight-forward tips learned from decades of pediatric practice on how to prevent this problem. This important work will be of help to all parents in keeping their offspring healthy for life."

—J.A. Stockman III, MD
Professor of Pediatrics, Duke University Medical Center
Past President, American Board of Pediatrics

"A fun, easy to read common-sense guide for parents and grandparents wanting not only to avoid obesity in their children but also to help children acquire lifetime good nutrition and exercise habits. The advice is basic, old-school pediatrics written in a style that speaks to Dr. Eden's years of experience as a pediatrician guiding pediatric patients and parents."

—Gerald M. Loughlin, MD, MS
Chairman, Department of Pediatrics, Weill Cornell Medicine
and Pediatrician-in-Chief, New York-Presbyterian Hospital

"*Obesity Prevention for Children* reflects 40 years of clinical practice by an unusually astute, highly competent, and compassionate clinician with a particular interest in nutrition and obesity. Of great value is Dr. Eden's anecdotal examples of obese patients and their families which offers useful new information on obesity. This book is a must have for all parents and professionals dealing with obesity."

—Philip Lanzkowsky, MD, ScD, FAAP
Professor of Pediatrics, Hofstra-Northwell School of Medicine

"This practical, no-nonsense book, written by an experienced pediatrician and leading expert on childhood obesity, will be useful for every parent. The real-life stories are drawn from Dr. Eden's extensive experiences as a practicing pediatrician, and breathe life into his advice and provide encouragement."

    —Michael Weitzman, MD

        Professor of Pediatrics, Environmental Medicine, and Global Public Health at the New York University School of Medicine

"Dr. Eden's philosophy is easy to put into practice and involves the entire family so that all can benefit from his wisdom. As parents and pediatricians, we must strive to prevent childhood illnesses, especially those that will impact our children as they become adults. Kudos to Dr. Eden, a world-class physician, mentor, and all-around great guy, for helping our children stay fit and trim!"

    —Claudio Sandoval, MD

        Professor of Pediatrics, New York Medical College Attending Pediatric Hematologist Oncologist, Maria Fareri Children's Hospital

"Finally, practical advice to prevent obesity from starting—the only way to really address the obesity epidemic. A must read for parents today. This text combines the latest scientific nutritional studies with simple, practical advice to prevent obesity—all with a conversational-style text. What more could parents ask for?"

    —Michael J. Pettei, MD, PhD

        Associate Professor of Pediatrics, Hofstra-Northwell School of Medicine Director, Division of Pediatric Gastroenterology and Nutrition, Cohen Children's Medical Center of New York, Northwell Health Co-chairperson, Nutrition Committee, American Academy of Pediatrics, NY Chapter 2

OBESITY
PREVENTION
FOR CHILDREN

BEFORE IT'S TOO LATE
A PROGRAM FOR TODDLERS & PRESCHOOLERS

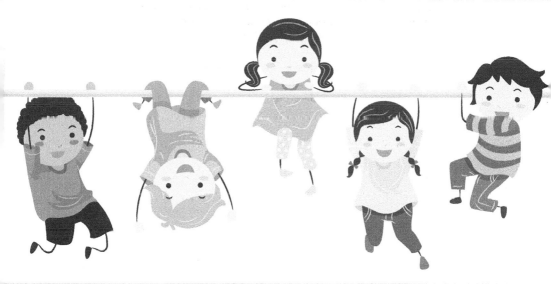

FEATURING RECIPES AND MEAL PLANS

ALVIN N. EDEN, MD
SARI GREAVES, RDN

Obesity Prevention for Children
Text Copyright © 2016 Alvin Eden, M.D.

Library of Congress Cataloging-in-Publication Data is available.
ISBN: 978-1-57826-647-0

BOOK DESIGN BY CAROLYN KASPER

Printed in the United States
10 9 8 7 6 5 4 3 2 1

CONTENTS · · · · · · · · · · · · ·

PART III: MEAL PLANS FOR TODDLERS AND PRESCHOOLERS

INTRODUCTION

I N 1975, I PUBLISHED MY first book, *Growing Up Thin*, which addressed the problem of obesity in children. It was a huge success and received a great deal of publicity. Yet despite these efforts, 40 years later children are fatter than ever.

So what happened during these past 40 years?

1. More and more meals are being eaten in "fast-food" establishments.

2. Portions sizes are now larger.

3. Besides TV, we now have computers, cell phones, and tablets for children, all of which increase sedentary time—what I call "S.O.B. Syndrome" (Sitting On Butt).

4. Physical education time in schools has become more limited.

5. More safety issues associated with outdoor play, such as increased automobile traffic and fear of abduction.

In truth, the obesity problem actually dates back to the 1950s, during which period food production in the United States dramatically increased. Starting at that time, billions of dollars began being spent to produce and market high-density, high-calorie foods at a relatively low expense to the consumer. According to a *New York Times* report in August 2008, sugar consumption rose by nearly 33 percent due to the use of high fructose corn syrup alone. The average American was now eating 1.8 more pounds of food each week.

The statistics are frightening. About 6 percent of Americans were obese in the 1950s, rising to 25 percent by the 1970s. Today, the figure is about 35 percent. The prevalence of childhood obesity has also increased significantly—two- to three-fold—just in the past few decades. An early childhood longitudinal study of over 7,000 children published in the *New England Journal of Medicine* (July 2014) showed that over 25 percent of children entering kindergarten were either overweight or obese. These overweight and obese kindergarteners were four times as likely to have remained obese into the 8th grade, as compared to children of normal weight entering kindergarten. In fact, nearly two out of every three children who enter kindergarten obese will remain obese as teenagers; in turn, most of those will end up obese as adults. In other words, if your child starts kindergarten overweight or obese, he will be at an extremely high risk of remaining that way throughout childhood and beyond.

The current childhood obesity epidemic is in large measure due to the modern high density, high calorie sugar-laden diet. This, together with a more sedentary life style explains why today we have so many overweight and obese children (and adults). Yet the consequences of developing obesity as a child are well known: in addition to reducing an individual's overall lifespan, other negative results include the development of type 2 diabetes, elevated cholesterol, orthopedic problems, sleep apnea, and a variety of psychological/social problems brought on due to a lack of self-esteem and self-worth. Obese children are also more likely to be bullied and socially isolated.

What's worse, this epidemic of childhood obesity has remained with us despite massive efforts to halt it in place—or at least slow it down. Up to this point, the majority of our efforts have been unsuccessful, if well intentioned. The answer is obvious. Having been a practicing pediatrician for over 40 years now, with a particular interest in this subject, my experience (as well as that of many other physicians caring for obese children) strongly suggests that the treatment of both school age and adolescent obesity is almost always unsuccessful. Sad though it is to say, the treatment of obese school-age children and older teenager is usually doomed to fail.

The basic problem is that neither the pediatric community nor the parents of young children are taking early onset obesity seriously enough. It is often difficult to convince parents that during the first five years of a child's life there even *is* a problem. In truth, most pediatricians do very little to encourage parents toward lowering the risk of obesity in their very young children. It is of interest to note that, within the recommendations of the American Academy of Pediatrics "Bright Futures" program, none of the well child visits for children ages 2–4 years list either diet or nutrition as a priority.

What has become increasingly obvious to me is that the only way to make any inroads into the problem of childhood obesity is to *not to let it happen in the first place*. In other words, *prevention*—rather than treatment—is the key to success.

And that is what this book is all about.

Quoting from an editorial in *JAMA Pediatrics,* August 2013, in an issue devoted to childhood obesity: "Targeted interventions aiming to prevent obesity *before* it is established . . . may offer the potential to break the vicious cycle of obesity." The article goes on to say, "Infancy and the early childhood years are "sensitive" periods of growth and development, presenting the opportunity to either reduce or increase the risk of later obesity." Based on the results of many studies on the treatment of childhood obesity, the authors conclude that parental motivation plays a strong role in predicting the effects of childhood obesity intervention. Further, family-based interventions have been found to be most effective, and the earlier they are started the better.

This book is my next—and hopefully final—attempt to help level the playing field for the next generation of infants, toddlers, and preschool children. It is my firm hope that they will not have to face the physical and emotional consequences and health risks of obesity as they grow up. If I am successful, even with only a few readers and their children, I will consider my legacy to be complete.

When the entire family works together, intervention becomes much more successful. There is nothing magical about this program. It is simple, straightforward, and safe. It is based on my long experience as a practicing pediatrician, as well as the most recent scientifically proven studies about childhood obesity. Learn to take an active role in your children's health. Protect your child from ever having to worry about being overweight or obese.

A NOTE FROM THE AUTHOR

As I have stated in all my previous books, I firmly believe in the equality of the sexes. Unfortunately, the English language does not provide any graceful word to substitute for "his" and "her," or "he" and "she." Therefore, I have again decided to alternate the pronouns used to describe gender. Please remember that these pronouns refer to your child, even if he or she is of the opposite sex. Similarly, 'you" refers to both mother and father (with one exception, and that being any discussion related to breastfeeding).

PART I

. . . .

TODDLERS (1–3 YEARS)

Chapter 1
OVERVIEW

THE TODDLER YEARS (children ages 1–3) are among the most important and challenging years you will face as a parent. It is during these crucial two years that lifelong eating and exercising habits be established. Your child's brain is also growing rapidly. Speech, understanding, and motor coordination begin to develop and expand at a tremendous rate. If done right, your child will be on his way to a happy, healthy, and productive life, protected against becoming overweight or obese. However, if you do things wrong, you risk jeopardizing his future health and well-being.

To complicate matters, it has been my experience that many parents either do not recognize that their toddler is overweight or obese, or else they choose to ignore what is obvious to others. Parents sometimes believe that their little child is leaner than she actually is.

"Dr. Eden, I am very upset. At her third birthday party, Amanda was called fat by her 6-year-old cousin. Now, I know that she is not thin, but surely she is not fat." In fact, by measuring her BMI I determined that Amanda was indeed obese. She was also visually obese to everybody—except her mother. After pointing this out to her, Amanda's mother fully accepted the facts and promised to do something about it.

A recent article published in *Pediatrics* confirms this: in a review of 80,000 parents questioned, two-thirds of those surveyed underestimated the weights of their children ages 2–19. Over half the parents of overweight and obese children underestimated their weights. Of particular interest was the finding that parents of 2–5 year olds were most likely to *underestimate* the weight of their children. The sooner these sorts of false impressions are identified and corrected, the sooner necessary actions can be taken to remedy the problem.

It is extremely important that you monitor your toddler's weight at every visit to her physician. Your toddler's physician will determine her percentiles by using her height and weight until age two, after which they will use the BMI (body mass index), which will be discussed in detail later on. This percentile tells you whether your child is of normal weight, overweight, or obese. Falling below the 85th percentile is considered normal weight; between the 85th and 95th percentile is overweight; and if the child is over the 95th percentile, then he or she is, by definition, obese.

While you may not realize that your toddler is already overweight, her percentile will prove it. Knowing your child's percentile is critical in the prevention of childhood obesity. If it starts edging up toward the 85th percentile, you have the chance to take action to prevent her becoming overweight or obese. If your toddler is already over the 85th percentile, immediate changes in diet and physical activity are required to slow down her weight gain and lower her percentile into the normal weight category. If your toddler is already over the 95th percentile, it's certainly not good news—but don't worry; you still can do something about it.

It's been my experience that many of the mistakes made by parents feeding their toddlers occur simply because they just do not know any better. Despite this, faulty feeding practices can have lifelong adverse consequences, including paving the way to "early-onset" obesity. (We'll be discussing these errors shortly, as well as the dos and don'ts of proper nutrition, in order to help you avoid trouble.) Early-onset obesity, the obesity that starts during the toddler and preschool years, has been shown to be much more difficult to treat than "late onset" obesity, the obesity that develops during the teenage and adult years. The point I want to emphasize to parents of toddlers is that what you do now will largely determine whether your toddler is destined to grow up with the serious physical and psychological dangers of childhood and adult obesity. This principle will be repeated and emphasized throughout this book. It is our basis for success in eliminating the epidemic of school-age, adolescent, and adult obesity.

Chapter 2
THE GENETICS OF CHILDHOOD OBESITY

THERE IS ONE IMPORTANT FACTOR related to obesity that you and your child cannot do anything about, and that is your genetics. You did not have a choice of parents and neither did your toddler. And let's face it, obesity *does* run in families. A child born to two obese parents has an 80 percent chance of also becoming obese. If one parent is obese, there is a 50 percent chance that that child will become obese. With two thin parents, the odds go down to 10 percent.

Notice a pattern? It is well known that body types run in families. Just go to Disneyland and watch families walking along together. Each family member is usually similar in build. The shorter, rounder body types—the endomorphs—usually have more trouble losing weight and maintaining normal weight than the taller, leaner body types—the ectomorphs.

But why?

Some of us find it very difficult to maintain a normal weight, while others have no problem staying thin. Why do some people put on weight easily and others eat all they want and never gain an ounce? That is the $1,000,000 question, and is yet to be fully answered. I call this the "X-factor"—the mysterious reason that some folks burn up their calories more slowly and less efficiently than do others.

FINDING THE X-FACTOR

One long-standing theory implicates the center in the brain relating to appetite. Dr. Norman Jolife, one of the pioneers in nutrition and obesity, named this center the "Appestat." Perhaps the appestat is preset higher in some families, causing them to have larger, genetically predetermined appetites. There is no question that some young children are voracious eaters while others have much smaller appetites.

Dr. Joseph Majzoub, the chief of endocrinology at Boston Children's Hospital, was the lead author of a recent paper that may be the answer to the X-factor question. In this study of mice, a gene was located in the mouse brain that actually controlled how quickly and efficiently calories were burned. When that gene was deleted, those mice gained weight much more rapidly than the mice that were left with that gene intact (with both groups consuming the same number of calories and exercising similarly). In addition, the investigators determined that the mice with the deleted gene also had greatly increased appetites later on in life.

One new theory comes from a study involving both humans and mice, which demonstrated that gut bacteria—the billions of bacteria in the intestine that help digest food—may play a role in determining if a person becomes fat or thin. Preliminary results, based on transferring gut bacteria from identical twins, one obese and the other thin, into mice, showed that the mice who received the gut bacteria from the obese twin became fat, while the mice getting the gut bacteria from the thin twin remained lean. If these results are duplicated and confirmed it will be an important advancement in our understanding of the genetic component of obesity—one that could lead, in time, to a possible treatment for obesity.

More research will be required before we can determine whether humans also have a gene or sequence of genes that control how quickly calories are burned up. If we do, then we will be on the way toward solving this problem. However, as this is still a ways off in the future, we must look for other, more immediate solutions.

Whatever the reason or reasons, we know that there is a strong genetic component in obesity. Identical twins raised apart from birth have adult weights that are very close to each other. One large-scale investigation found that, as adults, only 2 percent of identical twins differed in weight by more than 12 pounds. On the other hand, 50 percent of fraternal twins who were raised apart had adult weights more than 12 pounds apart. Adopted children have been shown to have weights closer to their biological parents than to their adoptive parents, further proof that genetics play an important role in the development of obesity (or lack thereof).

> *This reminds me of two very obese parents who came to see me with their 3-year-old girl for the first time; the child was complaining of a persistent cough. As I started to examine Susie, I remarked how happy I was that she was not overweight, since obesity seemed to run in their family. I wanted to know what they were doing to keep Susie so thin and fit. Her mother answered, "Absolutely nothing at all," which came as a surprise. It wasn't until a bit later that I found out that Susie was adopted when she was 2 years old!*

Dr. Albert Stunkard, a pioneer in obesity research who sadly passed away recently, conducted some landmark obesity studies in Denmark. His results conclusively established that some people are just genetically predisposed to getting fat, and that genes play a major role in body weight. He compared the body weights of identical twins, some who were adopted and some who were not. His study found that regardless of whether the twins were raised together or apart, each identical twin's BMI was almost the same.

Even if your family is "high risk" or genetically predisposed to obesity, there is no reason to be discouraged. It does mean that you will have to work that much harder to make certain that your toddler does not become overweight or obese. The rewards are unquestionably worth the effort. The obesity cycle *can* be broken—and we will help you do it. As Dr. Walter Willett, chairman of the Nutrition Department at the Harvard

School of Public Health, said in the *New York Times*, July 21, 2014: "Genes alone cannot account for the huge increases in obesity we've seen around the world."

> *I recall discussing proper nutrition with the parents of Josephine, a lovely 15-month-old, during their first visit to my office. Both parents were morbidly obese and I was worried about their "high-risk" child. They told me that, unfortunately, just about everybody in their family was overweight, going back to their grandparents. They seemed resigned to the fact that Josephine had little chance of avoiding what they called "the family curse."*
>
> *I spent the next 30 minutes telling them how wrong they were. Despite the family history, there was no reason to give up. I explained that, while yes, genetics is an important part of the equation, if they started now, I was certain they would raise a normal weight child. They did not look very convinced. I then told them that studies have shown that fat people raise fat dogs, and that has nothing to do with genetics.*
>
> *The good news is that when last I saw 10-year-old Josephine, she was of normal weight. Besides that, both parents, while still far from slim, had lost a good deal of weight themselves since that first encounter.*

By following the obesity prevention program laid out for you in this book, even the obesity-prone or "high-risk" toddler can be kept at normal weight. It works in my office—it will work for you and your toddler as well!

Chapter 3

WHAT WILL CHANGE WHEN MY BABY BECOMES A TODDLER?

T HERE ARE A NUMBER OF factors that come into play around the time your baby graduates from infancy and enters toddlerhood (after his first birthday). These may result in a too-rapid rate of weight gain, starting him down the slippery slope to childhood and adult obesity. Understanding and anticipating these changes can help you keep your child on the road to long-lasting health and normal weight.

SLEEP

Many toddlers today simply do not get enough sleep. The "terrible twos" often start before the child's first birthday, at which point negativity becomes the order of the day. Bedtime becomes a battle of wills between parent and toddler—a battle that you must strive to win, as a proper sleep schedule is vital to the prevention of childhood obesity.

A number of studies have demonstrated a definite relationship between the amount of sleep a person receives and obesity; namely, the less sleep, the more obesity. The specific reason or reasons for this association are not clear; it may be that fatigue leads to less activity, or it may be due to more time being available for eating, or it may be due to some appetite regulating hormones produced during sleep. It may even be a combination of all three.

The Albert Einstein College of Medicine in the Bronx, NY, conducted a study in which they followed over 1,800 children from age 18 months to 5 years. They concluded that children with short sleep duration (defined as less than 10 hours per night) at age 5 were twice as likely to be obese at age 15 as compared to children with longer sleep duration (defined as at least 12 hours of sleep per night).

Similarly, a recent investigation by the University College of London concluded that toddlers who get too little sleep tend to eat more. The study included 1,300 British families with young children; the amount of sleep was measured at 16 months of age and diets were calculated when the toddlers were 21 months old. The results showed that the toddlers who slept less than 10 hours a day consumed 10 percent more calories than the toddlers who slept more than 13 hours a day. The authors suggest that shorter sleep schedules may disrupt the regulation of appetite hormones.

It is very clear that the lack of sufficient sleep increases the chances of childhood and adult obesity. The American Academy of Pediatrics recommends at least 12 hours of sleep per day for children from birth to 2 years, and at least 11 hours per day for children 2–5 years old. Instilling proper sleeping habits has become part of winning the battle against obesity (see Chapter 11 for more information).

DECREASED APPETITE

As your child's rate of growth slows down at around 1 year of age, so too does their appetite. Many toddlers become what parents call "picky" or "finicky" eaters. In a large toddler study, half the mothers of children ages 19–24 months reported picky eating in their toddlers. Yet many of these finicky eaters actually gain weight too rapidly. The problem with many toddlers is this: toddlers drink excess calories and gain too much weight, despite a decreased appetite for solid foods.

"Dr. Eden, what's wrong with Amanda? She used to be a wonderful eater, but now she refuses all foods. Thank God she drinks gallons of milk and apple juice."

It is perfectly normal for a toddler's appetite to decrease at this age. If you think about it, it makes perfect sense. After 1 year of age, everything normally slows down, including weight gain and height increase. Appetite is no different; it is for this reason that doctors counsel parents never to force their children to eat. (Believe us, he won't starve!)

Ellen Satter has written about the concept of division of responsibility in foods, and we agree with her. Parents are responsible for what foods are being served and when, and children are responsible for how much they eat. We further advise parents *not* to allow their toddler to consume huge quantities of milk and juice, as this will only lead to obesity and iron deficiency. It will also diminish whatever small appetite he has left for nutritious solid foods. We advise you to restrict the daily amount of milk to a maximum of 24 ounces, which gives him more than his daily calcium requirement. Cut down juice intake to a maximum of 4 ounces a day preferably in the morning, and encourage water every chance you get the rest of the day.

FOOD DEMANDS

By 15 months of age, most toddlers are capable of feeding themselves table foods and drinking from a "sippy cup" without help. They rapidly develop the fine motor skills needed to scoop food and raise a spoon to their mouth without spilling the liquid all over. (They also become very skillful in throwing food and spitting it out at you!)

As your toddler grows, he will also become more assertive and demanding as he is better able to indicate his likes and dislikes.

> As one delighted parent put it: "You know, doctor, every day Mark is becoming more of a person." Another upset mother asked me what to do about her 2-year-old, Jonathan: "He doesn't talk much but when I put any food on his plate that he doesn't like, he smiles and throws the plate on the floor." That was a tough one for me to answer. I didn't advise her to send him out for adoption . . . but I thought about it.

This can be an exciting time for you and your toddler, as he expands his vocabulary and understanding. He can now ask for the foods or drinks he likes and reject the ones he dislikes. You now have a big decision to make. Do you give in to his every demand to avoid a battle? Or do you act like a responsible parent, interested in his health and well-being?

If you respond favorably to too many of his demands for cookies, candy, juice, soda, and all the other so-called "treats," you will be doing your toddler a great disservice. Not only will these non-nutritious high-calorie "treats" diminish his appetite for healthier foods, it will establish eating patterns that will continue as he grows up, inevitably leading to extra, unwanted pounds. We may be repeating ourselves, but *children develop their eating habits early on, and once established they are very difficult to change.* Not to mention, if you give up your dominant role as parent now and surrender to his demands for high-calorie, high-sugar snacks and treats, you will surely find it next to impossible to take a stand later on when his faulty eating habits are even further established.

You are not depriving your toddler of anything important by limiting his "junk foods." In fact, it's just the opposite. By standing firm, you will save him from a lot of grief later on, including obesity and high dental bills. Don't feel guilty when you say no and stick to your guns. He will thank you some day—and even if he doesn't, you'll still have done the right thing.

Food as Reward

I strongly advise that you never use food as a reward. There are plenty of other ways to reward your toddler. Negotiating with a toddler should not include food bribery.

However, in my experience this is a common practice for parents looking to exert control over unruly children. "If you are a good boy and eat your vegetables, I'll give you a cookie" is not the way to go. This early association between food and good behavior only starts a vicious cycle, leading to all sorts of eating disorders later on, including obesity. I worry about the toddler whose parents allow unlimited "empty" calories to reward good behavior, just to avoid temper tantrums.

I recall one exception to this rule. Many years ago, one of the toddlers in my practice loved broccoli. It was his favorite food. Need I say more?

I am not suggesting that candy or cookies be banned completely, or forever. There is no evidence to suggest that a slice of cake or dish of ice cream is harmful. But save the "treats" for special occasions.

Food Acceptance

As pointed out previously, a child's preference for the taste of sweet drinks and foods starts early on. Compounding this is that the acceptance of other, non-sweetened foods is not immediate, and may occur only after a number of exposures to those foods. The current Pediatric Nutrition Handbook of the American Academy of Pediatrics states that it may take 8–10 exposures to a particular food before the toddler accepts it. The previously discussed study from the University of Leeds also showed that toddlers who did not like vegetables usually took 5–10 exposures to the particular food before eating it, after which that particular vegetable was accepted without difficulty.

The mother of 2-year-old Danny was skeptical when I told her about this study, but she agreed to give it a try with broccoli. A couple of weeks later she called to report that, believe it or not, it had started working at the tenth and final try. Danny was now eating broccoli without any problem. She said, "I was about to call you to tell you that your system doesn't work, but lo and behold! It's like a miracle."

A study involving 332 children 6–38 months of age from the UK, France, and Denmark concluded that exposing the infants and young toddlers to vegetables early on resulted in their eating more vegetables as compared to a group who was offered vegetables at an older age. An interesting study that was conducted in British schools and homes found that when young children were given very small portions of a vegetable each day for 14 days, dislike often turned to like.

Offering new, healthy foods should feel like a game rather than like punishment. The point is to start offering vegetables as early as possible, as this will increase the odds of your child becoming a regular, happy veggie eater. The American Academy of Pediatrics' Nutrition Handbook reported the findings of one study indicating that many parents are not aware of the lengthy (albeit normal) course involved in achieving food acceptance in toddlers. 25 percent of mothers reported offering new foods only 1–2 times before deciding whether the child liked it, and 50 percent made similar judgments after 3–5 times. Touching, smelling, and playing with new foods (as well as spitting it out) are all normal. These are exploratory behaviors before the toddler finally accepts the particular food.

The moral of this story is not to give up too soon when offering nutritious foods to your child. It may take some time, but he will gradually learn to accept and actually enjoy the good stuff—believe it or not.

Chapter 4
SUGAR, JUICE, AND MILK

WHY DO CHILDREN ENJOY SWEET tasting foods so much? There is some evidence that the human desire for sweets is innate: a painting found in a cave in Spain, estimated to be 20,000 years old, shows a Neolithic man stealing honey from a beehive. We know that taste buds are already present and functioning in 4-month-old fetuses. One study even reported that, at 5 months of fetal life, the swallowing rate of the fetus increased after a sweet solution was injected into the amniotic sac. Newborns similarly exhibit positive responses to sweet solutions while remaining indifferent to salty solutions.

However, while the taste for sweetness may be genetic, the taste for overly sweetened drinks and foods is definitely acquired. Infants will drink plain water without a problem, but if offered sugar water first, they will then refuse to drink plain water. Your job as a parent is to prevent your toddler from developing a taste for high sugar drinks and foods. If you are successful, it is far less likely that your child will ever become overweight or obese.

SUGAR

The Centers for Disease Control and Prevention Division of Nutrition published a study in *Pediatrics* in February 2015, evaluating the sugar content of U.S. commercial infant and toddler foods. Of particular interest is that 41 of the 79 meals consisting of mixed grains and fruits contained added sugar. In fact, they found that over 35 percent of the calories in the food itself came from the sugar. 32 percent of toddler dinners and the majority of toddler cereals, fruits, and desserts contain added sugar. With this in mind, it is a good idea for you to carefully check the food labels when buying toddler foods. Remember, it's best to limit the amount of sugar your child eats each day.

A large-scale recent study of 2–5-year-olds published in *Pediatrics* in August 2013 showed a clear relationship between the consumption of soda and fruit drinks (those that were not 100 percent fruit juice) and obesity. At age 2, about 10 percent of the toddlers were drinking over 8 ounces of these sugary drinks a day, with percentages only increasing over the next 3 years.

A recent longitudinal analysis of sugar-sweetened beverage intake further confirmed this relationship. 1,189 newborns participated in the Infant Feeding Practices Study II in 2005–2007, with a follow-up at age 6 in 2012. The results demonstrated that the children who consumed the sugar-sweetened beverages during the first 2 years had higher odds of being obese at age 6 than the children who did not drink those types of beverages.

Despite all the sugar hiding in their diet, it has been my experience that many parents go out of their way to sweeten the foods they serve their toddlers—especially vegetables. The thought is that this will make the vegetable more palatable to a picky toddler. This is a bad idea for the following two reasons: first, the extra sugar with its extra calories is obviously unhealthy, and second, it just plain does not work. A very recent study from the University of Leeds in the UK titled "Often and Early Gives Children a Taste for Vegetables" concluded that there was little difference in the amount of vegetables eaten over time between those toddlers fed a basic artichoke puree as compared to those toddlers who were given a sweetened artichoke puree. The bottom line is that sweetening a vegetable will not make a significant difference in the amount your child eats. I can only hope that this helps to dispel the popular myth that a vegetable's taste must be masked in order for a child to eat it.

You will find out—if you haven't already—that toddlers can be stubborn, manipulative, negative, and even nasty as they fight for what they want. The "terrible twos" are a normal developmental milestone. The entire world revolving around him and nothing else seeming to matter is a characteristic of the toddler years. Sad to say, some of us never grow out of it.

Nobody said it would be easy. But if you are sufficiently motivated, you *can* do right by your toddler. In short, put your foot down when your child demands sugary snacks and drinks. We are firm believers in negotiation and compromise, but not at the expense of your child's health and well-being.

> *This reminds me of a mother describing her toddler as follows: "There is no question that Alex will become a lawyer, defending and acquitting murderers. He's already figured out how to get me to give in to his pleas for huge quantities of apple juice. If he can already manipulate me at age 3, what chance will a jury have?"*

But what if your child isn't genetically predisposed toward obesity? You may be less inclined to fight with them over sugary snacks and beverages. However, while a diet high in sugary drinks, snacks, and foods certainly does lead to obesity, it is unhealthy for another reason, as well.

We are referring here to the so-called "empty calories." Let us consider a toddler who consumes about 1,500 calories per day. With this calorie allowance, she should eat foods that contain essential nutrients for optimum health. These include vitamins, minerals, essential fatty acids, amino acids, complex carbohydrates, and fiber. The greater the number of "empty" calories in her diet (those calories lacking in these essential nutrients), the more likely the total diet will not supply all her needed nutrients. Candy, soda, sweetened fruit drinks, cookies, cakes, and other highly sweetened foods add very little nutritious value, despite technically providing a daily calorie allotment. Hence, these are called "empty calories." Because those highly sweetened foods taste so good, toddlers, if given the chance, will consume large amounts of extra "empty" calories they don't need, and less of the nutritious foods that they do need.

To put the (hopefully) final nail in sugar's coffin, the American Heart Association has unequivocally linked excess sugar to heart disease. It is important to remember that most of the sugar we eat comes from foods like cookies, cakes, candies, and cereals (only about a third of our average sugar consumption comes from soda and sweetened drinks). Many of these sweet-tasting foods are also very high in fat; donuts are a perfect example of this.

It is vital that our daily sugar intake be cut down dramatically in order to prevent both obesity and heart trouble later on. But enough about sugar for the moment. By now, I am sure you've got the message. While the occasional "treat" is okay, it's best to eliminate the sugary drinks and snacks from your toddler's daily diet.

JUICE

Most parents consider 100 percent juice a "natural" healthy nutritious drink for the toddlers. And it *is*—provided it's not consumed in excess. That 100 percent apple juice you so confidently give your child hides some secrets:

- 1 cup of apple juice contains 24 grams of sugar and 114 calories.
- It takes 1 pound of apples (or two cups of sliced apples) to make one serving of juice.
- 1 cup of sliced apples contains 11 grams of sugar and 57 calories.

Whole fruit is a much better choice for your child than fruit juice, for three reasons:

1. Whole fruit contains less calories and a lot less sugar.
2. Whole fruit contains more fiber.
3. Whole fruit satisfies hunger more quickly than juice.

Speaking of apple juice, apple juice has been shown to be responsible for a greater percentage of fruit juice intake than all the other fruit juices combined, according to a recent survey conducted by the Health and Nutrition division of the Centers for Disease Control and Prevention (published in the October 2015 issue of *Pediatrics*).

The Dietary Guidelines Advisory Committee states that no more than one-third of the total recommended daily fruit group intake should come from fruit juice. The remainder should come from whole fruit in order to meet the requirements for vitamins, folate, and potassium. It is clear that an important obesity prevention principal is to limit daily juice intake.

In a prospective observational analysis published in *Lancet* about the relationship between the consumption of sugar-sweetened drinks and childhood obesity, the findings demonstrated that children increase their chances of becoming obese by 1.6 times with each additional cup of sugared beverage they drink each day. Excessive fruit juice replaces other nutritious foods in a toddler's diet, including milk, whole grains, meats, fruits, and vegetables. This can result in a diet with inadequate intake of protein, fat, calcium, vitamins, iron, and zinc (it may also cause diarrhea, although apple juice appears to be the main culprit in this). Since it is easier for your toddler to drink juice than to eat a piece of fruit, they consume more of it. This in turn causes the calories from too much juice to add up quickly, translating into extra, unneeded pounds.

> *I recall the mother of a 21-month-old who could not understand why her Janet was so overweight. She said, "Dr. Eden, Janet is such a picky and finicky eater. She hardly eats anything." It turned out that plump Janet drank well over 32 ounces of apple juice each day.*

It is clear that an important obesity prevention principal is to limit daily juice intake. The American Academy of Pediatrics recommends limiting daily juice intake to 4–6 ounces. My recommendation is a maximum of 4 ounces a day.

As a reminder, I am discussing 100 percent pure juice, and *not* fruit *drinks*, which should *never* be offered to your child. Many studies show a clear relationship between fruit drinks and soda consumption and obesity in young children. Good old plain water is the best drink of all, not only to help prevent obesity, but for the overall health of your child. If your toddler learns to drink water to quench his thirst rather than a sugary flavored drink, he will be a lot better off in the end. We may sound like a broken record, but instilling proper eating and drinking habits early is the key to the prevention of obesity later in life.

MILK

Milk is certainly a healthy food and is essential for supplying calcium to a toddler's diet. The problem is getting the right amount. There is an old saying, "A quart of milk a day keeps the doctor away." Not true; the Committee of Nutrition of the American Academy of Pediatrics recommends 2 cups of milk per day for a toddler (a total of 16 ounces). This fulfills all her calcium requirements.

Just as with juice, too much milk crowds out other needed foods, making it more difficult to achieve a well-balanced nutritious diet. Between the ages of 1 and 2 years, the Academy of Pediatrics recommends that a toddler drink whole milk. After age 2, the recommendation is to switch to low-fat or skim milk, and I agree. However, if a toddler is overweight or obese, I suggest starting low-fat milk at 1 year of age. This is an easy and effective way to cut down on some calories.

> *I remember a mother asking me about this and questioning why I wanted such a drastic change. "Dr. Eden, you want to put Joseph on 2 percent fat free milk? That seems such a drastic switch from whole milk, which is 100 percent fat." It was then that I explained that whole milk has about 3½ percent fat, not 100 percent fat.*

Chapter 5
FOODS

THE TODDLER YEARS ARE NOTORIOUS for poor nutrition, over-nutrition, or both. There is a normal physiologic decrease in appetite for foods and increased juice and milk consumption. During the so-called "well-baby" visits your infant makes to your pediatrician or family physician, you were given specific instructions about the types of baby food. But after 1 year, the doctor visits become less frequent, and a child's diet is not monitored as carefully. Often, parents are told to switch from baby foods to more adult-type table foods, along with switching from breast or formula to whole milk.

This results in large changes in the toddler's diet, often very unhealthy ones. If your family's meals are well balanced and nutritious, your child is a lucky kid. Sad to say, the typical American family eats a diet that is too high in calories, saturated fat, cholesterol, salt, and refined sugar. This is the wrong diet for everybody, including your toddler. The type of diet you feed your toddler now becomes the diet he will continue to eat as he grows up. Not only is this type of diet too high in calories, but it can start your toddler down the slippery slope toward heart problems later on in life. At a recent American College of Cardiology meeting, research was presented showing that about one in every three children between ages 9 and 12 in the United States have borderline or high cholesterol levels. Other studies have demonstrated that many first- and second-grade children already have elevated cholesterol levels and high blood pressure.

Let me tell you about Luis, age 3. I first saw Luis in my office when he was brought in by his two obese parents. They were concerned about a rash; I was concerned about Luis's weight. He was already markedly obese, just like his parents. They didn't seem to worry about his weight; however, when I explained to them that if they didn't start making changes in their son's diet and exercise soon, he would become at high risk for both high blood pressure and an elevated cholesterol level.

My lecture seemed to make an impression. When I saw Luis six months later, he was still overweight, but his weight gain had slowed down and his blood pressure was normal. Besides making changes in his diet, his parents were concentrating on keeping Luis physically active. Unfortunately, many parents are not this compliant and cooperative.

Again, let me repeat—eating habits are instilled *early*. Once established, they are hard to change. If the diet you feed your toddler is too high in calories, he *will* become overweight. This gives him a greater chance to become an overweight or obese school-ager, who in turn becomes the obese teenager.

Here are some shocking statistics from the current Pediatric Nutrition Handbook of the American Academy of Pediatrics:

1. Between 28 and 33 percent of toddlers do not consume any fruit on a given day.

2. Between 18 and 20 percent of toddlers do not consume vegetables on a given day.

3. The vegetable most commonly eaten by toddlers is French-fried potatoes.

Data from the Infant Feeding Practices Study II and the 6-year follow up study suggest that this infrequent intake of fruits and vegetables during the toddler years is associated with infrequent intake of fruits and vegetables at 6 years of age and beyond. Further proof of this comes from data analyzing the school lunch programs that require distribution of one fruit or one vegetable at every lunch, and the tremendous amount of wasted food that has resulted from this practice as many children refuse the fruit or vegetable. The conclusion is that many school-age children are not accustomed to eating fruits or vegetables, making the early introduction of fruits and vegetables even more important.

I strongly encourage you to offer your toddler servings of fruits and vegetables every single day so that they learn to not only accept them as a regular part of the diet but to learn to *enjoy* eating them. As previously pointed out, some vegetables take a large number of encounters before they are accepted.

Your whole family should be on the so-called "prudent" diet, a heart healthy diet low in calories, The Dietary Guidelines for Americans encourage children to consume adequate amounts of fiber-rich fruits and vegetables and whole grain products. These guidelines advise that the diet provide 30 percent of the calories from fat while using low-fat milk, beans, lean meats, poultry, and fish. We recommend that you cut down on fatty red meats such as bacon, sausage, hamburgers, and steak, and instead offer chicken (not fried) and veal instead.

It is also very important that your toddler be offered fish at least two times each week. The Food and Drug Administration and the Environmental Protection Agency of the federal government now recommend a minimum of two servings a week of low mercury seafood such as salmon, shrimp, cod, tilapia, and light canned tuna. This latest advisory discourages your child from eating high mercury fish such as shark, swordfish, king mackerel, and tilefish from the Gulf of Mexico. This is the diet that the American Academy of Pediatrics recommends for all children starting at age 2, and it is the type of diet that we strongly advise you follow. Not only is this a healthy, nutritious diet but it is also lower calorie than the typical Western diet.

Chapter 6
TASTY AND NUTRITIOUS MEAL PLANS

Y OUR CHILD IS ON A tasting adventure from the moment solid foods are introduced. Making meals look and taste appealing increases the chance of good nutrition from childhood into adulthood. Treat your toddler or preschooler as a miniature adult by encouraging them to try the same types of foods that you are eating at meals. If you keep portions to about a quarter of an adult portion size, there is no need to count calories or worry about over-feeding your little one. If your child wants to eat more, you can always give her seconds, like another tablespoon of vegetables or the other half of a piece of fruit. Don't worry about your toddler "cleaning their plate" at every meal. Building a balanced diet involves offering repeated opportunities for your child to try new foods.

The following are general guidelines, specific diet plans, special recipes, and between-meal snacks that follow guidelines of the American Academy of Pediatrics. They are nutritious, delicious, and tailored not only to help prevent your little child from becoming overweight but also to help him develop proper eating habits and preferences that will go a long way toward ensuring that he never need fight a battle with obesity. It will also protect him from heart trouble as an adult by keeping both blood pressure and cholesterol levels within normal limits.

Offer three small meals and two snacks a day to support growth, energy, and nutrition. Use every meal and snack as a "pit stop" for mixing and matching different food groups. Young children may need to eat five to six times a day to optimize diet variety because their small stomachs don't hold much. Aim for them to get a variety of nutrient-rich foods over the course of a week.

As a parent, you serve as a diet "GPS," leading your child down a path of healthy food choices and eating habits. Serve designer meals featuring a wide variety of colors and textures. Purchase or cut foods into interesting shapes and arrange it attractively on a plate. For example, you can find crinkle-cut butternut squash "fries" or zucchini "spaghetti" at some grocery stores. Serving the same food in different forms—for example, cooked carrot coins and raw carrot sticks—can improve your child's acceptance of new foods

Offer new foods at the start of a meal when your child is hungriest. Prepare a dish for the whole family, with the only variation being size and texture—smaller portions and softer textures for your toddler or preschooler—and serve it alongside a familiar food that your child regularly consumes. Allow hot food to cool down and cold food to warm up a little before serving; avoid meals served at extreme temperatures.

A small flavor boost can enhance taste, but avoid going overboard. Heavily spiced, salted, buttered, or sweetened dishes may prevent your child from experiencing the natural taste of Mother Nature's healthiest foods. Young children also tend be more sensitive to flavors than you are, and may reject heavily seasoned foods.

Choose the right plate for easy portion control. Have no time to weigh, measure, and calculate portions? As a guide, offer one tablespoon of every food served (about the size of a poker chip) for every year of age. A child-sized, sectioned plate is an easy way to introduce toddlers and preschoolers to healthy portions. Available for purchase online, the 8-inch USDA *Choose MyPlate* has four sections for different food groups. The Protein and Fruits segment measures ¼ cup, and the Vegetable and Grains section measures ⅓ cup. You can also send a healthy message about portion control by decreasing the size of your plate. Try switching from a dinner plate to a salad plate or look for vintage plates that are smaller in diameter. (Research on adults has shown that by switching to a 10-inch plate from a 12-inch plate, you eat 22 percent less.)

Grains to grow on. Choose whole grain tortillas, breads, cereals, and pastas. Select brands with short, understandable ingredient lists made from a variety of whole grains including organic whole wheat, barley, millet, oat, brown rice, whole corn, and spelt.

Pump up the iron. I have been particularly interested in the subject of iron for many years, and have conducted research and published extensively in the pediatric literature regarding the relationship of iron deficiency and impaired mental and psychomotor development. You can think of iron as a guardian angel that helps protect your child's physical and mental growth. Iron is an essential mineral that is needed to make hemoglobin, the oxygen-carrying component of red blood cells. Red blood cells deliver oxygen throughout the body. Without enough iron, the body's tissues and organs don't perform at peak level. Iron deficiency may lead to learning and behavioral problems.

While an iron-fortifying multivitamin provides insurance from your toddler's unpredictable eating, remember that supplements are not magic substitutes for a balanced diet. "Food first" is the best way to satisfy your child's daily iron needs. The most easily absorbed iron—called heme iron—is found in animal proteins. The plant form of iron—called non-heme iron—is not as well absorbed, but still offers valuable nutritional benefit. Heme iron helps absorb non-heme iron, so pair them together at mealtime. Create kid-friendly meals and snacks, such as whole grain turkey roll-ups, beef and bean tacos, or hummus-dipped chicken bites. (Refer to the meal plan section on how to create these fun iron-rich food combinations!)

Here's a quick checklist of iron-rich foods to include in a balanced meal plan:

- Heme iron–rich "M-F-P" foods: meat, fish, poultry (and eggs)

- Non-heme iron-rich food: beans, hummus, tofu, leafy green vegetables (turnip greens, kale, broccoli) and enriched grains (with 10 percent or more of the daily value for iron)

Count on Vitamin C. Vitamin C-rich foods such as potatoes, broccoli, and citrus fruits increase iron absorption. Good match-ups include: iron-fortified oatmeal with bite-size pieces of oranges, strawberries, or kiwi; hummus with red pepper strips; or iron-enriched pasta with steamed broccoli "trees."

THINGS TO REMEMBER

The act of eating is a skill. Your child is still learning to chew and swallow efficiently, and may gulp food in a hurry to get on with playing. The risk of choking on chunks of food is especially high in young toddlers; chewing with a grinding motion isn't learned until they reach about four years of age. Make sure anything you give is mashed or cut into small, easily chewable pieces.

Practice caution with the following foods:
- Hot dogs (slice lengthwise and then cut into small pieces)
- Whole cherry tomatoes, raw carrots (cut into quarters)
- Whole grapes (cut into quarters)
- Whole nuts (ground or processed into small pieces)
- Chunks of peanut butter (it's fine to thinly spread on a cracker or bread)
- Avoid raw cherries with pits
- Avoid hard candies, jelly beans, gummy bears
- Avoid raw celery

Chapter 7
PHYSICAL ACTIVITIES FOR TODDLERS

PARENTS SOON FIND OUT THAT most toddlers are absolute dynamos. As they learn to walk, run, and climb, they develop a great desire to get around—to explore and learn about their environment. That being said, not all 1–3 year olds are energetic and adventuresome. Some toddlers are pretty sedentary and placid, quite content to just sit around and spend their time watching TV and eating snacks. Studies have shown that many 3–5 years olds spend over 30 percent of their waking time just sitting around.

In one of my previous books, I called this type of behavior SOB. syndrome (Sitting On Butt syndrome). If your toddler fits into this category, you'd better do something about it now.

"You know, Dr. Eden, Jenny is a perfect little angel. She's happy to sit in her high chair watching TV for hours at a time," the mother of a two-year-old told me during her visit. Jenny was far from the thinnest child in my practice. I explained that if nothing was done to change Jenny's behavior, sooner or later she'd find herself in real trouble. We discussed active intervention, including restricting TV and encouraging physical activity.

Regarding the active toddler, there is always the question of safety— you cannot leave a toddler on his own. He must be protected from hot stoves and electric wiring, and from tumbling down a flight of stairs. Outdoors, you will be faced with a different set of threats to his well-being. All of these variables must be considered when planning and supervising your toddler's play time.

But there *is* such a thing as being *too* safety conscious. Toddlers are sturdy and well-engineered, and are very capable of absorbing falls, scrapes, and scratches without permanent damage. By restricting him from moving around and getting his share of bumps and bruises, you will discourage him from exploring and learning—and from burning up calories. Furthermore, you will be encouraging a sedentary life style, something you do not want for your child.

Your job is to provide your toddler with a variety of safe opportunities for exercise. Without a lot of encouragement on your part, the sedentary toddler will spend more and more time sitting around, staying out of trouble and inevitably, gaining more weight than he should. You should encourage and motivate him to use his body and find a joy in movement that will remain with him as he grows into an active healthy school-ager and teenager.

EXERCISE

At its most recent meeting in Washington, D.C., the U.S. Department of Health and Human Services spelled out its physical activity guidelines. It highlighted various interventions that can be used to increase physical activity in children and adolescents ages 3–17 years. Their report was well meaning, but in my opinion, misses the point. As far as prevention of childhood obesity is concerned, starting interventions at age 3 is much too late if you want to make a real dent in the current epidemic.

There is a direct relationship between exercise and obesity at any age, including the toddler years. Many overweight toddlers actually take in *fewer* calories than their thinner playmates, counter to conventional wisdom. All things being equal, you would expect a child who eats less to weigh less. In many cases, all things are *not* equal, because of:

1. The genetic X-factor that we discussed earlier, where the "high risk" child simply burns up calories less efficiently

2. The overweight or obese toddler becomes less active than his thinner colleagues, and therefore burns up fewer calories.

Physical activity of any kind burns up calories. The more active your toddler, the more calories burned up over the course of a day. Each day counts; just a few extra calories burned via exercise every day will make a huge difference, especially for the "high-risk" or already overweight toddler. A recent large-scale study published in the *International Journal of Obesity* found that taking your children out to play several times weekly is an easily attainable, immediately effective goal that might prove useful in the prevention of childhood obesity. In other words, make it your business to take your little child outside to play as often as you possibly can. When you think about it, this makes perfect sense. Indoor play restricts your child from active physical activity and calorie burning. Remember: outdoor play should not be something reserved for warm sunny days—many parents believe that just about every day should be an outdoor day!

We are reminded of many popular "old wives' tales" that many parents believe; namely, that taking a child outside on a cold winter day will lead to pneumonia. This is complete nonsense. Pneumonia and other respiratory illnesses are usually caused by viral infections (and rarely by a bacterial infection). They are not caused by cold weather. The weather should not interfere with outdoor play, with the possible exception of hurricanes, tornados, and blizzards.

Regardless of what came first, the obesity or the lack of exercise, it really makes no difference—if your toddler is already overweight, there is no reason to panic. You still have time to correct the problem, but only if you increase his daily physical activity (in addition to modifying his diet). When it comes to regular daily physical activity, I do not believe in a "hands-off" policy. Don't assume that she will get as much exercise as she needs. In fact, most obese toddlers have a tendency to be less active; carrying around extra pounds makes it more difficult to run and jump around easily.

As discussed earlier, safety issues are of course important. But instead of curbing and discouraging your little child from running, jumping, tumbling and hopping simply because of your concerns about injuries, figure out a way to give her the space and time to exercise in a safe environment. If you don't have a backyard, regular visits to a playground can substitute.

TV

Once your child becomes a toddler, television—the great pacifier—now comes into the picture full-time. There is little question that running after an active toddler all day long is hard work. Even the most devoted parent needs an occasional break. Plopping your little child in front of the TV can do just that. As your toddler learns to understand words and talk, he will start to take a greater interest in watching TV, especially if you or any other older siblings spend long hours glued to the screen. It is estimated that 90 percent of toddlers regularly watch TV. In addition to TV, many toddlers already use mobile devices (such as tablets).

"Finally, I can get a little work done without having to worry that he will get into big trouble." I often hear sentiments like this from mothers who use the TV as a babysitter. I can certainly sympathize with them, and I do not think that such mothers should be arrested for child abuse. But they are taking the easy way out—and odds are, they won't be the ones paying for their little parenting shortcuts.

The point we want to make is that TV time should be limited. The American Academy of Pediatrics recommends *no* TV for the first two years of life, but we think that this is a bit drastic. My advice is no more than one hour of TV a day, spent watching educational programming rather than cartoons. It is a very bad idea to allow your toddler to spend hours on end staring at the TV screen; a toddler who is allowed to sit quietly watching TV for hours each day is very likely to grow up with the same habits, which will inevitably lead to overweight and obesity.

Encouraging safe, active play instead of TV is good insurance against obesity. If a toddler watches more than two hours of TV per day and sleeps less than 12 hours a day, he has a six times greater chance of becoming overweight or obese compared to toddlers who watch no TV and sleep at least 12 hours a day.

One morning, one of my patients brought in her 2½-year-old son David for his regular checkup. We talked about his sleep pattern. She reported that David always fell asleep in his bed, watching cartoons. I told her in no uncertain terms to move the TV set out of his room and to figure out a way to remove the cartoon channel permanently. I told her that David would have to find another way to fall asleep.

GAMES AND ACTIVITIES

For 1–2 year olds

The following are some specific suggestions to help your young toddler become strong, agile, and coordinated, while burning up calories to help prevent obesity. (In the case of the already overweight or obese toddler, these activities will help him get back to normal weight.) These activities and games are age-appropriate for both boys and girls. They do not require expensive or elaborate equipment, but they *do* require a commitment on your part—your time and effort every single day.

Push and pull toys: Cars and trucks, often with noises and sound effects built in, make for a fun activity, and not only for little boys—my daughter is an example of a little girl who found this activity wonderful. These toys encourage lots of physical activity, and are useful for both small and large muscle development. It gives your child the opportunity to exercise in his make-believe world, which is great for both physical and emotional development.

Balls: Balls of various sizes and shapes, all large enough not to be swallowed or choked on, are terrific toys for a toddler. He can learn to throw and even catch it if it's large enough. I know of no toddler who doesn't enjoy kicking a ball, chasing it, and kicking it again. However, I strongly suggest that this remain an outdoor activity. (A mother once called me to complain about her 2-year-old who kicked a ball and broke her window from inside her house. All I could think of to say was, "There might be a soccer scholarship in his future.") Learning to throw, catch, and kick a ball helps build hand and eye coordination and agility. If you have a future Federer or Messi at home, this will give them a good start!

Crawling games: Excellent for indoor playtime, crawling games provide for large muscle development. You can use your imagination to figure out ways to make it fun; my favorite was simply cutting out the side of a large cardboard box and creating an indoor playhouse for my children to play in. Crawling around on the floor with your youngster can be great fun for both of you—although it will be a little harder on your knees than his! It's also a good time to hug and snuggle (we call it our "rainy-day" activity!)

Roughhouse activities: This is an all-time favorite of ours. As with all the physical activities we encourage, you don't require special equipment or expensive apparatus; all you need is a blanket or pad. There are no rules, simply make them up as you go along. Anytime of the day is fine, except for the bedtime hours when too much vigorous exercise will interfere with sleep. This type of all-over activity involves all of your toddler's muscles, which is great for burning up excess calories. These gentle roughhouse activities are also good for his emotional well-being. You are giving him your full and undivided attention as you have fun together, which is so important for building up his self-worth and self-esteem. Note: it's a good idea to stop frequently during your wrestling and tickling for rest periods and a glass of water.

Hop and skip games: This is another fine parent-child activity that you can do both indoors and outdoors, though it is best done outside. Toddlers rapidly develop the ability to skip, and you will no doubt start to wear you out if you try to keep up. The problem is figuring out a way to stop them! Chances are that an expert and experienced hop-and-skip toddler will not have a weight problem.

Outdoor play yard: This is ideal if you have a yard available for personal use, be it yours or a neighbor's. A public playground with proper safety equipment is just as good. Make it your business (and the business of any childcare agency or babysitter you employ) to take your toddler outside as often as possible. It is unfair and unhealthy to keep a toddler cooped up inside all the time. The greater his opportunities to run, jump, and climb, the stronger and healthier he'll be, and the less likely it is that he will be obese.

Slides and climbers: In backyards and playgrounds, these are great sources of fun-filled physical activity that contribute toward agility and coordination. Obviously, these are to be used only under careful supervision.

Four-wheeled vehicles: No, not an automobile; these toys are powered by your toddler's feet! The toddler can sit on or straddle these vehicle and move around, exploring his world from a new vantage point. He'll use up a lot of calories in a short period of time, and it's good preparation for his first tricycle.

Hide and seek/Ring around the Rosie: These are two time-honored favorites that are great fun and terrific exercise.

For 2–3 year olds

While all of the suggestions for children ages 1–2 are just as viable for children ages 2–3, once your child gets a bit older, new opportunities for growth and exercise become available.

Between 2 and 3 years of age, toddlers begin to enjoy rhythmic play, like dancing or riding a tricycle. More active games become possible, involving all sorts of vigorous, independent activity—pulling and pushing wagons, playing with toy trucks and wheelbarrows.

This is a good time to begin helping your child to develop sports activity skills. Golf, tennis, and skiing might still be a bit beyond them, but it is not too early to think about swimming, soccer, wrestling and playing catch.

Swimming: This is an ideal skill and sport that most toddlers love. I encourage teaching toddlers to swim, but as they often have no fear of the water, accidents are possible. A toddler should never be allowed in the water on her own; rather, she should only swim under strict supervision with you or with another adult in the water with her.

There are organized swimming programs available to teach your children to swim, including many YMCAs. Swimming is one of the "carry-over" sports, meaning an activity that can continue all through life (as opposed to baseball or football, sports that stop after graduation). These "carry-over" sports should be cultivated early on, for future health and maintenance of normal weight.

Soccer: This is another excellent activity for children of this age group. I can think of nothing that is more fun and better exercise at the same time; that soccer is also a potent calorie burner is the icing on top. It develops great coordination, speed, and endurance, and builds to other sports later on, including tennis and basketball. Even the less active toddler will learn to enjoy soccer with sufficient encouragement and perseverance on your part.

Throw and Catch: By 2 years old, toddlers can throw a ball, sometimes fairly accurately. Catching a ball, however, is not that easy. The key to success is practice, practice, practice. Don't worry; you will tire long before your toddler. This activity improves the hand and eye coordination that is so important for many sports, including baseball, basketball, and tennis.

Wrestling: This was a favorite physical activity with my two children when they were toddlers, and even once they got older, we still had loads of fun—and you will, too. A good wrestling match builds up strength, stamina, agility, and balance and gets rid of plenty of extra calories. I also seem to recall there being a lot of tickling and laughing besides the wrestling in our house!

Becoming skillful in any physical activity or sport helps to build a child's self-esteem and self-confidence. It also makes it more likely that the young child will continue with that particular activity as he grows up. All of this is healthy, but more importantly, it serves as insurance against becoming overweight or obese later on in life.

We would like to share with you data from a most interesting Australian community-wide intervention program, published in the

Journal of Clinical Nutrition (2010), which was aimed at reducing obesity in early childhood. This large-scale community effort was conducted over a 4-year period (from 2004 to 2008), during which time 12,000 children, 0–5 years of age, and their families, were targeted with the following four messages:

1. Daily active play
2. Daily water and fewer sweet drinks
3. Daily fruits and vegetables
4. Less screen time (TV and DVD)

The entire community was involved, including schools, the press, churches, health fairs, radio, and TV-trained early childhood professionals, lectures and conferences. This massive intervention program was successful in reducing the prevalence of childhood overweight and obesity in the 2–3½ year olds, as compared to a neighboring community where this targeted intervention was not carried out. The conclusion of the study was that it is possible to prevent your toddler from becoming overweight or obese.

I believe that you do not need a 4-year community intervention plan to be successful. My program will do the job just as well—and you don't have to move to Australia to do it!

Remember, the goal is to raise a happy, healthy child who never will have to suffer the physical and emotional consequences of childhood and then adult obesity. Following my plan will protect your precious child from growing up overweight and obese—and a big part of that plan is instilling in your child a genuine skill for and appreciation of active physical play.

. . . .

PART II

PRESCHOOLERS (3–5 YEARS)

Chapter 8

OVERVIEW

Y OUR CHILD HAS NOW GRADUATED from toddlerhood and entered into her preschool years. She is either normal weight, overweight, or obese. If she is normal weight, congratulations! The diet and exercise program that you have been following has been successful (or maybe you're just lucky, and she is genetically programmed to remain fat free). If your preschooler is already overweight or obese, you had better get busy and do something about it. You still have the opportunity to prevent her from suffering a lifetime of obesity, with all its medical and psychological consequences.

The years between ages 3 and 5 are particularly important in terms of the prevention of obesity. Many children accelerate their weight gain during this period. One recent study demonstrated that over 50 percent of obese 3–6 year olds remained obese as adults.

ADIPOSITY REBOUND

One of the reasons that this period is so critical for the development of obesity is *adiposity rebound*. First described in 1984, this refers to a phenomenon observed around a child's fifth or sixth year, in which their BMI first falls, and then quickly rises. Early adiposity rebound is an important risk factor associated with an increased risk for adolescent and adult obesity. Not allowing your preschooler to become overweight or obese will automatically move her into the late obesity rebound, which is protective against obesity later on in life.

Since it was first described, clear and consistent associations have been demonstrated between earlier (before age 5) rebound and overweight and obesity in teenagers and adults. Two recent studies demonstrate this phenomenon. First, an Australian study which enrolled 341 4-year-olds and followed them for the next 4 years. The early rebounders—those whose BMIs rose before they were age 5—were shown to have a significantly increased risk of being overweight or obese by age 6 or 7, as well as being more likely to be overweight or obese as adults. Second, a New Zealand study of 458 children followed from birth to age 26, demonstrated that 69 percent of early rebounders (before age 5) were found to be overweight or obese as adults.

I recall discussing adiposity rebound with the parents of 4-year-old twins, who were both overweight. After a few minutes, I realized that I wasn't getting through to them and so I stopped trying to explain the phenomenon and simply told them that all it meant was that gaining too much weight during the next 12 months was the worst time of all to put on extra pounds. It would result in putting both boys at a very high risk for permanent obesity for the rest of their lives. That seemed to make an impression!

For reasons like adiposity rebound, the treatment of childhood and adolescent obesity is usually ineffective and often unsuccessful; we have known this for many years. A recent large-scale review and meta-analysis of 15 separate studies measuring the impact of diet and exercise interventions in obese school-agers and adolescents revealed that none of the 15 studies resulted in any meaningful long-term weight loss. And even when treatment has been successful, the relapse rate is well over 90 percent. Quoting Dr. Seema Kumar, a pediatrician at the Mayo Clinic's Children's Research Center: "The money lies in prevention." Healthy eating and adequate physical activity must start early, so that it may become second nature for your child. This is the core premise of this book: that *early life prevention* is the best way—if not the *only* way—to finally control the epidemic of childhood obesity.

And there *is* hope of success. A most recent study, published in *JAMA*, demonstrated that there *has* been some success in actually reducing the prevalence of obesity in preschool-age children. This federal survey found a slight drop in the obesity rate in 2–5 year olds as compared to the previous survey. Of particular interest is that the same survey showed no change in the obesity rates in older children and adults. Of course, only time will tell whether this reported decreased rate of obesity in toddlers and preschoolers will continue. Nevertheless, these results suggest that we may well be successful if obesity prevention is started early.

GENETICS

Childhood obesity must be considered the number one health problem for parents in the United States, even above smoking and drug abuse. Yet in our experience, many parents either do not understand the consequences or are not worried enough about early childhood obesity. There are some parents who still believe that it is healthy for a child to be overweight. How often do we hear, "What a lovely chubby little girl"?

Folks, nothing can be further from the truth. Hospitalizations of obese preschoolers continue to increase due to obesity-related conditions, such as diabetes, fatty liver, asthma, pneumonia, and gallbladder disease. Other serious problems associated with obesity include obstructive sleep apnea, hypertension, and depression. Large increases in weight during this particular period of your child's life (3–5 years) have been conclusively shown to lead to adult obesity. Preventive strategies must be started now. As pointed out in the 2013 position paper of the Academy of Nutrition and Dietetics, active participation by the parents is necessary for a child's health in general, much less the prevention of childhood obesity. Weight goals must be monitored closely in order to be successful in preventing childhood obesity.

New research has further confirmed the fact that obese school-aged children already show signs of future cardiovascular problems. In a study carried out at Leipzig University in Germany, the obese children studied were found to have significantly higher cholesterol and triglyceride levels than the normal weight children observed. Furthermore, the obese group had lower levels of "good" cholesterol (HDL) and higher levels of "bad" cholesterol (LDL), as well as higher blood pressure. Finally, using echocardiograms the researchers found that on average the obese school-agers had thicker heart muscle than the normal weight children, a finding that would point to cardiovascular trouble if seen in an adult. Quoting from the lead author of this study, Dr. Norman Mangner: "We do not know if these changes are reversible with weight loss or how they will impact future cardiovascular disease in these subjects."

Beyond the adverse physical consequences, preschool obesity leads to psychological and social problems that will only increase in frequency and severity as the overweight child grows older. Dr. Albert Stunkard, in his book *The Pain of Obesity* cites a 1960s survey that illustrates this, in which a group of children were shown photographs of other children, some of whom were normal weight, some disabled, and others obese. The children were asked to pick out those they would like to have as friends. Almost invariably, they picked the obese child last. Sad to say, prejudice and social stigma against the obesity is widespread, and it starts with children.

If your preschooler is already overweight or obese, you had better get busy doing something about it. You still have the opportunity to prevent her from suffering a lifetime of obesity, with its many medical and psychological consequences. The emotional toll can be painful; if not now, then surely later on at school. Many obese preschoolers are clumsy and may be shunned to the sidelines by their peers during games and team activities.

That being said, we do not recommend a weight *loss* program for the obese preschooler (absent the rare exception). Rather, the goal is to slow down weight gain to achieve normal weight. But the longer your preschooler remains overweight or obese the more difficult it will be to slim her down. And it *can* happen before you realize it; as early as age 3, a large number of obese preschoolers have already developed "high risk" factors for heart disease. Many exhibit elevated blood pressure, high cholesterol and triglyceride levels and inflammatory markers, putting them on a clear path to severe problems such as heart attacks and strokes later on in life. In other words, this is serious business.

The good news is that even if your preschooler is overweight or obese, you can still turn things around, and I will tell you how to do it. Don't buy into the "baby fat" myth—the idea that overweight or obese little children naturally shed their pounds and slim down later on. It simply does not work that way—quite the opposite, in fact. By age 3, the food patterns, eating habits, and physical activities that have been promoted and developed during infancy and toddlerhood begin to solidify and take hold. Unless you intervene now and make the necessary changes in her diet and physical activity, the "baby fat" will become "permanent fat," and your child will be well on her way to having a constant weight problem as she grows up.

There is no such thing as "spontaneous" slimming down. It is for this reason that, barring very rare exceptions, we do not recommend a weight *loss* program for an obese preschooler. Rather, the goal is to slow down the weight gain to achieve normal weight. The rate of weight loss can't be gamed or hurried; in other words, the longer your preschooler remains overweight or obese, the more difficult it will be to slim her down.

If your child is overweight, don't look for a miracle cure. Rather, accept the challenge to remedy the situation. Every month you continue to allow her to eat more than she needs of non-nutritious foods and drinks, and every month you postpone and neglect instilling good exercise habits, you only lower her chances of growing up with a normal weight. The time to act is now.

Some years ago, a very overweight mother brought her obese 4-year-old in for her checkup. Before I could say one word, she said, "Dr. Eden, please don't lecture me about Katherine's weight. Everybody in my family is overweight, going back two generations. We're cursed. There is nothing we can do about it. It's genetic and not our fault."

I spent the next 30 minutes trying to convince her otherwise. I wasn't very successful, but I kept on trying. It took a while to get her to change her attitude. Happily, we were able to slow down Katherine's weight gain and she has since become a competitive swimmer. Following my family-oriented diet and exercise program worked for Kathy, and while it was a difficult journey, it was well worth the effort.

GETTING STARTED

Easier said than done, I hear some of you saying. There is no question that many of us are playing on an uneven playing field. The genetic factor in obesity cannot be ignored; some people just do not burn off calories as efficiently as others, and this often runs in families. I am reminded of an old expression from poker: "You play the hand you're given." You may not *like* the hand you're dealt, but you have no choice. You just do the best you can, and believe it or not, sometimes you can win the whole pot.

The program that I am discussing—the program that I have been teaching in my office for many years—has been successful in preventing childhood obesity, even with "high-risk" families (families with many obese members). Don't get me wrong; it may not be easy. It has its ups and downs and it takes a lot of work on your part, but if you are sufficiently motivated you *can* do it, even if genetics aren't on your side.

To begin, we must first determine whether your child *is* obese, and if so, how far advanced the issue is. Many parents don't realize that their child is obese, thinking instead that she is "pleasantly plump." Others consider their normal weight child to be overweight.

Until recently, I had no standard definition of obesity. Now, with the use of the body mass index (BMI) I can point out to parents exactly where on the spectrum of healthy and unhealthy weight their child falls.

BMI is the most accurate measurement of your preschooler's weight status. It is a simple measurement, requiring only your child's weight, height, age, and gender. BMI readings are recommended by the American Academy of Pediatrics, to begin at age two at every well child visit to the doctor.

Using the BMI, a child will fit into one of three categories:

1. Normal Weight: Below the 85th percentile

2. Overweight: Between the 85th and 95th percentile

3. Obese: Over the 95th percentile

Your child's doctor can easily calculate the BMI and tell you your child's percentile. Unfortunately, a recent study determined that only 46% of the pediatricians who responded to a survey routinely calculated BMIs. I suggest you discuss with your child's physician if you are not given your child's BMI. These BMI percentiles offer the best way to track children's weight gain, especially those who are gaining weight too rapidly. Parents who are given accurate assessments of their child's weight status via BMI readings are more likely to make the weight-related behavioral changes in diet and exercise necessary to prevent overweight and obesity, and will usually do so sooner than if they were not aware of the BMI and what it means.

Let me give you an example: 4-year-old Andrew, the son of two obese parents, was doing fine. His BMI was at the 65th percentile and all was well, until he came in at age four and a half and his BMI had increased to the 80th percentile. We talked about it with Andrews's parents and they understood that changes needed to be made to keep him from becoming overweight (BMI over the 85th percentile).

There are times when the obesity-prone child can only be kept at a normal weight by consuming fewer calories than the non-obese-prone child; perhaps 10–15 percent fewer calories each day. At age 5, Andrew is now down to the 70th BMI percentile, and we are all happy.

As a frame of reference, a 4-year-old with a BMI over 17 is at the 85th percentile and considered overweight. If the BMI is over 18, it puts him at or over the 95th percentile, which defines him as obese. (This holds true for both genders; between the ages of 2 and 5, there is very little difference in the BMI between boys and girls.) Please see the Appendix at the end of this book for the BMI growth charts that your child's doctor will use to calculate the BMI percentile, based on the gender, weight, height, and age of your child.

As stated earlier, these preschoolers have minds of their own, and it can be difficult to get them to eat properly. Even at this young age, children have already begun to develop their own "lifestyle," complete with food preferences (often completely wrong), and their preferred level of physical inactivity (which may be unhealthy). If your child is already overweight or obese (remember the BMI) it is a good bet that she got there honestly, eating too much of the wrong foods and not being active enough. Just remember, your child has developed her "lifestyle" from you and not from anybody else. The buck can only stop with you.

I have found many parents who do not realize that they have an "ace is the hole" in the fight against childhood obesity, particularly during these formative years. Children have an innate desire to emulate their parents. Your child actively wants and tries to be "grown-up," and to her, "grown-up" means like Mommy and Daddy. Setting the right example is the key to just about everything, including preventing obesity. If you enjoy fruits and vegetables, chances are that in time your child will enjoy them too. If you drink water and not soda during meals, she will do the same. Believe me, she will not feel deprived of sugary drinks and high-calorie, non-nutritious foods if they are not part of her daily routine. By following the nutritious meal plans and snacks featured in this book, your child will have no choice but to eat what you offer at home (visiting Grandma is another story).

I recall meeting with the family of a 4-year-old boy named Joey. Both he and his father were both markedly overweight, and while Papa had pretty well resigned himself to being a fat person, he did not want Joey to have the same problem. We spent some time carefully outlining my diet and exercise program. Two weeks later, Joey's father called me, upset. "Dr. Eden, it is not working at all. Joey has been crying and nagging us about his food all day long. We end up giving him the stuff he shouldn't have just to get a little peace and quiet. What should we do?"

Putting on my Sherlock Holmes hat, I soon discovered that while Joey was being given the nutritious diet I'd recommended, Mom and Dad were still eating what they ate before.

To have any chance of success, everybody in the family has to eat the same foods. Thankfully, there is a happy ending to this story. Joey and his father came in three months later. Joey was grinning from ear to ear: "Me and my dad are on the same diet. We are getting into shape together and we are getting real strong!" One year later, Joey had grown 2 inches but only gained two pounds. Dad did not grow, but had lost 10 pounds. That made my day.

Chapter 9
FAT-PROOFING

THIS BRINGS US TO AN important concept, the matter of "fat-proofing" your house. This is a must if you are serious about preventing childhood obesity. It is the easiest thing in the world to do but most folks just don't do it. All it involves is a careful visit to your refrigerator and food cabinets, removing all the bad stuff—the soda, sugary drinks, chips, cookies, candy, and cake.

In terms of what you should do with all that food, you have three choices:

1. Go on a tremendous binge and eat it all yourself.

2. Give it away to a neighbor you are not particularly fond of.

3. Throw it away.

So, what should you keep, and what should you throw away? Besides the obvious sugar-laden snacks mentioned above, you should be looking to remove any obvious sources of empty calories. In terms of what liquids should be in your refrigerator, low-fat or skim milk, club soda, 100 percent orange juice, and water are your best bets—anything else is asking for trouble. (As stated earlier, we advise restricting juice to 4 ounces a day. Whole fruit is preferable to juice because whole fruit contains fewer calories and a lot less sugar, it increases your child's fiber intake all while increasing satiety. In other words, it satisfies hunger more effectively than juice, resulting in fewer calories consumed).

An occasional "treat" is perfectly acceptable, but should be reserved for special occasions like birthdays, special holidays, and once every leap year. A cookie or plate of ice cream is *not* poison; but by not having these so-called "treats" around the house, your child will have no choice but to eat and drink a nutritious, lower calorie diet. She will of necessity learn to accept and enjoy this type of diet, and more importantly, will *continue* to enjoy it as she grows up. These are the years when food preferences are established, and these do not change much later on.

> *I am a perfect example of this. My mother used to bribe me to eat my vegetables by offering me a black olive rather than a cookie or candy. To this day, I prefer salty foods rather than sweets of any kind. Fortunately for me, my blood pressure is okay!*

That's all well and good, you say, but what if *I* want to enjoy a soda with dinner or a bit of dessert in the evening? Can't I just keep the "bad stuff" out of my child's reach? Unfortunately, many parents think this way, without fully appreciating the damage this does to a child's chances of avoiding obesity. Restrictive feeding practices—not allowing the child to eat high-calorie, high-sugar foods and beverages that are on the table—have been shown to be an important risk factor in the development of childhood obesity. A study published in 2013 in medical journal *Childhood Obesity* showed that children whose parents used these restrictive feeding practices were 1.75 times more likely to be overweight or obese than children raised without these restrictive feeding practices. In order for my program of obesity prevention to be successful, the whole family must be in it together, with no exceptions.

As a side note: fat-proofing your house is a critical first step, but what about when the time comes for the family to enjoy an evening out? As compared to 30 years ago, eating out at fast food restaurants has increased 18 fold. The portion sizes of sodas and French fries have almost doubled. So what is one to do? Boycott McDonald's? No, simply use some judgment. How about a salad with the hamburger? How about fewer meals out? You can't fat-proof McDonald's, but you *can* bring that mindset with you wherever you go. The interesting thing is that your preschooler will learn quickly that there are two types of diet, the one she gets at home and the one she gets when eating out. And she'll be okay with that, as long as you are consistent.

Think of all this as getting rid of public enemy number one. By removing unhealthy food and drink from your home environment, you will be well on your way to raising a "fat-proof" child, a child who will be protected from ever becoming overweight or obese.

An out-of-town friend of mine brought his 5-year-old girl to see me for my advice about what he should do about her obesity (he himself was not overweight). I explained about increasing her physical activity and the type of diet she needed. He kept nodding in agreement until I got to the part about "fat-proofing" the refrigerator and he suddenly looked at me with the saddest expression I ever saw. He said, "But I love my Sara Lee cake with milk before I go to bed."

It can't work that way. In order for obesity prevention to work, everybody has to be in it together.

Chapter 10
TELEVISION AND SLEEP

As YOUR PRESCHOOLER BECOMES MORE and more aware of his surroundings, TV, particularly television advertising, will begin to be a big factor working against you in preventing childhood obesity. The influence of television on your child is profound; it is estimated that preschoolers watch 2–3 hours of TV each day. You will find it more and more difficult to help them maintain things like a healthy level of physical activity, or a low sugar diet.

There are three reasons why this "screen time" is responsible for much of childhood obesity. First, excessive TV watching reduces the number of hours left for physical activity, while increasing the consumption of calories (from snacking while watching television). Second, decades of research provide strong evidence that TV marketing is effective in establishing food preferences and requests. Children's TV programs have been particularly targeted, advertising nutritionally poor foods, especially sugar-sweetened drinks. And third, TV, especially in the bedroom, has been shown to be an important factor in reducing the amount of sleep the child gets each night.

> "Dr. Eden, my four-and-a-half-year-old Harold is very upset that we don't have any Coca-Cola in the refrigerator. He is always watching commercials on TV and asks for a coke each and every day. What should I do?"

This is an easy one to answer, but it *does* illustrate the pressure put on parents. Although the total sales of soda are currently slightly down, these drinks are still extremely popular. In 2012, Americans spent $65 billion on soda. A study published in the *American Journal of Clinical Nutrition* tested the effects of the consumption of high fructose corn sugar for two weeks on cholesterol and triglyceride levels. Quoting from the lead author Kimber Stanhope, "It was a surprise that adding as little as the equivalent of a half can of soda at each meal was enough to produce significant increases in the risk for cardiovascular disease." There is no question that the excessive intake of sugar is one of the major causes for the current obesity epidemic.

In fact, as food and beverage manufacturers continue to face increasing pressure to limit child-targeted marketing for sugar-sweetened beverages (chocolate milk and fruit drinks), there appears to be an increase now in parent-directed marketing of nutritionally poor foods and drinks.

Children's TV programs have been particularly targeted in advertising nutritionally poor foods, especially sugar-sweetened drinks. As food and beverage manufacturers continue to face increasing pressure to limit child-targeted marketing for sugar-sweetened beverages (chocolate milk and fruit drinks) there appears to be an increase now in marketing directed at parents. This was the finding of a recent study conducted by the Department of Pediatrics of the Geisel School of Medicine at Dartmouth College, Hanover, New Hampshire. This is of particular concern, since many parents misinterpret the nutrition and health claims in the advertising and actually believe that chocolate milk and sugar-sweetened drinks are healthy choices for their children. There is no question that substantial exposure to TV and its advertising is associated with a greater risk of overweight and obesity. By substantial, we mean over two hours per day. TV advertising continues to promote high calorie, low-nutrient foods and beverages. While I do not advocate a legislative ban on the advertising of junk food to young children, perhaps it is something we should seriously think about.

Of course, the problem is not limited solely to issues with targeted advertisements. Nor is it a problem specifically associated with your television set. Rather, they both illustrate a current trend toward less and less physical activity. A *New York Times* November 2015 article discussed the results of a study that found that a large number of 4–5 year olds, besides watching TV, are already using various devices such as computers and tablets to further their sitting on butt (SOB) syndrome. The American Academy of Pediatrics recommends limiting children's total screen time to no more than 1–2 hours of quality programming each day; we believe that, for preschoolers, 1 hour or *less* a day should be the goal. It goes without saying that no television set should ever be located in a child's bedroom; that practice has been shown in many studies to be a risk factor for obesity.

SLEEP

You would think that a child who slept less and stayed up longer would be burning more calories, and would therefore have less of a chance to become overweight. Wrong! Just the opposite is true. Poor sleep habits have been proven to be associated with childhood obesity. A study of preschool children found that those who slept less than 8 hours per night had an increased rate of obesity, and that the risk of obesity increased as sleep time decreased. Another study showed that children who slept less than 9 hours a night had 1.5 times the risk of being obese as compared to the children who slept more than 11 hours each night. A large-scale study of 7,000 3-year-old children concluded that sleeping less than 10.5 hours each night was associated with obesity at 7 years of age.

> *I recall discussing the relationship between sleep and obesity with the mother of 3-year-old Rebecca. "It doesn't make any sense, Dr. Eden. If Becky sleeps less, she will have more time to run around and burn up calories." I had to explain to her that it just doesn't work that way.*

The exact reason for the association of sleep and obesity has not been proven as yet, but the correlation itself is a fact. One very interesting study from the University of Illinois identifies sleep duration as one of the most important risk indicators for obesity. In another study, 329 parent/child pairs were evaluated to determine the greatest risk factors in developing obesity (the children were 2–5 years old). The results showed that there was a 2.2 times greater risk of overweight or obesity among children who slept 8 hours or less each night. The conclusion to be drawn by this investigation and others suggests that early childhood is the developmental period when sleep behavior, particularly lack of sufficient sleep, increases the obesity risk.

So: how much is enough sleep for your preschooler? According to the American Academy of Pediatrics, 2–5 year olds require a minimum of 11 hours per day. Children who meet this requirement lower their risk for obesity.

But some preschoolers are better sleepers than others. Many resist bedtime, figuring out all sorts of ways to stay up. This is perfectly normal behavior; just remember that adequate sleep is very important, not only in relation to obesity, but also to prevent fatigue during the day. Insufficient sleep can impair cognitive functioning and increase behavior problems. (The sleep deprivation I suffered during my pediatric residency days made me a pretty cranky fellow most of the time, according to my wife, but what is my excuse these days?)

A number of behavioral and environmental factors may contribute to inadequate sleep. Among the most common are:

1. Irregular bedtime and wake time

2. Inappropriate napping habits

3. Vigorous physical activity close to bedtime

4. Noisy or un-darkened sleep environment

5. TV in bedroom

(Again, we strongly advise that you never put a TV in your young child's bedroom. Not only will it act as a deterrent to a good night's sleep, but it helps lead the child to obesity, independent of the total TV viewing time.)

Your job is to create an environment conducive to ensuring sufficient sleep. This means a cool, quiet, dark room—without a TV in the bedroom. A dark room is very important; melatonin, the brain's neurotransmitter which regulates the sleep/wake cycle, is triggered by darkness and makes people drowsy. TV has a spectrum of blue light that is a potent suppressor of melatonin, and can easily disrupt sleep schedules. Try to avoid active physical activity for at least one hour before bedtime. I know that this is often difficult to achieve, but do the best you can. A regular bedtime routine or ritual is a must. How about a warm bath, reading a story, a good night hug and kiss, a tuck in, and lights out? The nature of the ritual is up to you; what is important is that you are consistent each night. Your preschooler *must* learn to fall asleep without you around.

I didn't follow my own advice when our son was 4. Often tired myself, I would lie down in his bed next to him to wait for him to fall asleep. Bad idea; I usually fell asleep first!

Chapter 11
FAMILY MEALS AND SNACKS

I T HAS BEEN MY EXPERIENCE—AND the conclusion of a number of studies—that the family eating together is crucial in preventing childhood obesity. Family mealtime is important for other reasons as well; it is the ideal (and often the only) time the family has to talk to each other, laugh together, bond together, and learn together. Busy schedules often make this difficult; nevertheless, try your best to eat together with your little child as often as you can, preferably eating the same foods. If a young child sees his parents eating a particular food, even asparagus or Brussel sprouts, he will be more likely to give it a try himself.

Whenever possible, it is a good idea to allow your child to serve himself, family-style, from a common bowl, teaching him age-appropriate portions. Using small plates can be helpful, to prevent overfeeding. If you serve the food, offer small portions, half of an adult portion (read more about portion size on page 68). You can always give him more if he finishes his plate and is still hungry.

Studies have demonstrated that frequent family meals are associated with a number of health benefits for children. One study from the University of Minnesota published in *Pediatrics* in November 2014 found that positive interpersonal dynamics such as laughing, having fun, talking, and listening resulted in children who were less likely to be overweight or obese. This was a two-year study of 120 families, using direct observation, data collection, videotaping, and interviews. Letting children play with their food and eat as much as they wanted—in a happy, stress-free environment—appeared to reduce the risk of developing obesity.

I was recently asked by the mother of 10-year-old Joseph and 4-year-old Louis how to handle the problem of feeding her two totally different children. "Dr. Eden, Joseph is thin and active and is a great eater. But little Louis is overweight, not very active, and is a picky eater. What can I do at mealtimes?"

That was an easy one; the food rules for both children should be the same. Healthy children, be they normal weight, overweight or obese, must all be offered a variety of healthy foods. There should be no "junk foods" in the house, and both children should sit down together for a regular family meal consisting of a variety of nutritious foods. As Dr. David Ludwig, the director of the New Balance Foundation Obesity Prevention Center at Boston Children's Hospital stated in a *New York Times* article on June 2014, "Everybody should be treated exactly the same; no junk food, no opportunity to feel unfairly singled out and stigmatized, and if the overweight child wants to snack it's fine to give him or her access to healthful snack foods. People don't binge on apples, because you fill up on them before a huge number of calories are consumed."

We completely agree with Dr. Ludwig. In our book on preventing infant obesity, *Fit from the Start,* we wrote about the possible reasons breastfeeding protects against obesity, involving a discussion of the internal cues for hunger and satiety, and learning to stop eating when no longer hungry. The same principle holds true for the preschooler. He should learn how not to overeat. The goal of a meal is not to clean the plate but rather to stop eating when full. One strategy is to serve your preschooler on small plates, offering small, child-size portions. If he finishes his plate and is still hungry, give him some more. What your little child must learn is to stop eating when no longer hungry rather than when the plate is empty or when you decide that he has had enough to eat. It is well known that the obese never allow the feeling of being satiated to interfere with finishing everything on the plate. In the section on toddlers, I emphasized creating a healthy eating environment; now, this is even more important. Let me repeat, it is essential to sit together with her and eat the same foods, with no distractions (such as you reading the paper or talking on your cell phone, or her watching TV, or playing with a tablet).

The result of a study recently conducted in Massachusetts is of great interest. It involved 121 families with 2- to 5-year-old children who had TV sets in their bedrooms. A 6-month intervention program was carried out, aimed at improving four specific household routines that had been shown to affect obesity:

1. Amount of sleep

2. TV in bedroom

3. TV screen time

4. Eating meals together as family

The intervention group was counseled about the importance of adequate sleep, having no TV in the bedroom, limiting the child's time spent watching TV, and eating meals together. In the end, while the intervention group was successful in eating together and reducing TV time, they were not successful in getting the TV out of the bedroom or increasing the daily amount of sleep.

Nevertheless, the intervention group evidenced lower BMIs than the control group, and that was with improvements to only two of the four household routines. For comparison, the program in this book includes all four of these household routines; so, if you are able to follow them all, your preschooler should have little risk of becoming overweight or obese. And the fact is that none of the four household routines are difficult to achieve.

A study reported in the *Journal of the American Dietetic Association* suggests yet another factor that may affect childhood obesity: the social-ization of children's eating at mealtime. The results demonstrated that 85 percent of the parents of preschoolers tried to force their children to eat more than they wanted, and 83 percent of the children were found to have eaten more than they might otherwise have. The techniques parents used were rewards, praise, or pressure tactics. These data reinforce our recommendations that a parent's job is only to *provide* nutritious foods, and the children's only job is to decide *how much* to eat at that meal.

FOOD PREFERENCES

There are two schools of thought about food preferences. Many health professionals take the position that getting rid of junk food and providing a nutritious diet will automatically result in the child developing healthy eating habits. On the other hand, many parents have difficulty with that, as they deal with the reality of children who seem to have been born with a dislike for anything healthy.

> *"It is hard to believe that my twins are so different," one mother told me. "Dr. Eden, Christine eats everything on her plate, including broccoli and asparagus, while Joseph refuses to taste any vegetable." Being in an especially jovial mood, I suggested that one of the twins probably belonged to another family. Fortunately, that mother had a pretty good sense of humor!*

We discussed food acceptance earlier, in the toddler section of this book. To recap, studies have shown that it usually takes 15–20 exposures to a particular unfamiliar or disliked food for it to be accepted by a young child. Most parents give up long before that, usually after only three or four times.

A very interesting study was just published in *Appetite from England* related to the subject of food acceptance and preference. It involved almost one hundred 12–32 month old children. An intervention was developed using games that featured unfamiliar but healthy foods that included looking at pictures of the food, feeling its texture, smelling it, and hearing its name. The targeted foods in the study were all healthy foods and vegetables. The results demonstrated a very clear impact on the children's willingness to try the targeted foods.

I remember the mother of a 5-year-old telling me that her son Nicholas loved pizza and asked for it every day. "Dr. Eden," she asked me, "what can I do about it?"

I explained to her that while pizza was not inherently bad, it certainly should not be eaten every day. I told her about a study published in Pediatrics *in 2015 about pizza, analyzing pizza consumption patterns in children, and estimating the impact on total calories, sugar, saturated fat, and sodium.*

The results showed that pizza consumption was significantly associated with higher daily calories, saturated fat, and sodium. The study further demonstrated that eating pizza as a snack or from a fast food restaurant has a greater impact on increasing calories. The authors of the study concluded that pizza consumption in children should be restricted and closely monitored, and I agree.

Getting back to little Nicholas, we agreed to compromise. Nicholas gets pizza twice a week and he seems happy with that.

We know that genetics does play a role in food tastes; it's related to sensitivity to sweet and bitter and even fat. We have also learned that the food preferences of parents do influence their children's choices in food. When I was younger, a common food bribe my mother would employ was to offer me a black olive, one of her favorite foods, in place of candy or other sweets. To this day, I have a preference for salty foods.

A most interesting study of twins published in the American Journal of Clinical Nutrition in 2014 from the Department of Epidemiology and Public Health of the University College of London England further confirms that both genetic and environmental effects were significant in establishing food preferences in children. The genetic effects appear to be more significant for fruits, vegetables, and meat, whereas the environmental effects dominated for snacks, starches, and dairy products. Again, nothing can be done about the genetic component, but plenty can be done about the environment.

JUNK FOOD

During the early years, your preschooler is almost totally dependent on you for every single bite of food she eats. Thankfully, it is not difficult to keep junk foods out of your own house.

But you don't live in a vacuum. Sometimes grandma is in the picture, or a babysitter or nanny, or the neighbors across the street with a house full of cookies and cake and candy. TV advertising remains a deadly enemy. But while food companies are free to promote unhealthy, obesity-producing stuff for your child on TV, you are just as free to say no to the ads, *and* to say no to your brainwashed child begging for whatever soda or candy was just on the screen.

> *A mother was complaining to me that her daughter Amy was very upset, because when she visited her best friend, she always was given chocolate cake and potato chips with Coca-Cola. I asked her if she did the same when Amy's friend came to visit. She answered, "No, I certainly do not." I was happy to hear that, and told her to explain to Amy that in our house we have different rules for our family, and that's the way it is going to be—no ifs, ands or buts.*

SNACK TIME

Let me share with you a food diary that 4½-year-old Amanda's mother brought to me at my request, because Amanda was quite overweight:

7 A.M.

4-ounce orange juice
Sugar puff cereal and whole milk

9 A.M.

2 chocolate chip cookies
1 cup whole milk

12 P.M.

Cream cheese and jelly sandwich
1 chocolate cookie
1 cup whole milk

2 P.M.

1 cupcake
1 cup fruit drink

3 P.M.

Ice pop

5 P.M.

½ bag of corn chips

6 P.M.

1 hot dog on roll
Mashed potatoes
Apple sauce
1 cup whole milk

8 P.M.

1 cup apple juice
2 chocolate chip cookies

You don't have to be a genius to see that Amanda's diet was much too high in calories and sugar. The ratio of treats to healthy nutritious foods was way out of proportion. After my usual lecture, Amanda's refrigerator and kitchen cabinets were "fat-proofed" once and for all, and a very unhappy Amanda started to eat a more sensible, healthy diet.

Kids love to snack, and Amanda was no exception. Studies have shown that at least 25 percent of calories children consume come from snacks and that most of the favorite snacks are "empty" calories, missing essential minerals and vitamins, while being high in sugar and fat. These are a major cause of overweight and obesity. Sad to say, snacking on unhealthy, high calorie/high sugar snacks is increasing. The University of North Carolina conducted a recent study with over 31,000 children, 2–6 years of age, and compared it to another large-scale study conducted in 1977.

Currently, young children average over three snacks per day, as compared to less than two snacks per day in 1977. Snacks are fine, but it depends on what kind of snack it is. If you offer healthy foods, rather than the sugary and fat-filled cookies and chips and sugary drinks, snacks are good—even encouraged.

Top 3 Tips for Healthy Snacking

1. Offer finger-friendly, bite-size food to encourage independent eating.

2. **Use snacks to fill in nutrient gaps.** Plan ahead by keeping food-group snacks handy. Space them at least two hours before mealtime; "pacifier snacks" eaten while standing in line at the supermarket or given half an hour before a meal may interfere with a healthy eating routine. Kids do better with a schedule, so try to serve meals at about the same time every day. Learning how to detect hunger and fullness is a skill that will make them less likely to overeat.

3. **Size matters.** Offer snacks in 4-ounce bowls for built-in portion control. Take and Toss Toddler Bowls with Lids or BPA-free small plastic containers are durable enough to use over and over (available at www.amazon.com). Snap-on lids help keep food fresh, and a ½ cup capacity makes them ideal for holding a variety of food-group combinations, such as yogurt and carrot sticks, whole grain crackers and hummus, or apples with cheese.

> *"You know, Dr. Eden, the only way Michael will eat any vegetables at all is if I bribe him with a chocolate bar. What can I do?" As discussed in the section on toddlers, never use food as a reward. Not only does it result in a diet with too many "empty" calories, but it starts a vicious cycle of equating junk foods with good behavior and feeling better when upset or depressed.*

Little children love sweets, even more than adults. There is a physiologic explanation for this; their taste buds are clustered. Children have as many taste buds as grown-ups, but since their tongues are smaller, the younger the child is, the more intense the flavors they experience. As Brian Walker, the director of Cornell University's Food and Research Laboratories Registry, said, based on the research of his group, "That's why little kids don't like bitter foods and really like sweet foods. The effect is magnified."

Nevertheless, as we've said time and again, the amount of sugar your child receives should be carefully monitored, and ideally come from healthier sources than candy and juice. Besides the extra "empty" calories in sugary foods and liquids, the frequent consumption of sugar can lead to dental cavities. Further, research has linked sugar consumption to other health problems, including high levels of glycerides and cardiovascular disease, as well as to type 2 diabetes.

Given free rein of the supermarket, what your preschooler would choose as her snack foods is no surprise. Let us repeat that it is very easy for your preschooler to become addicted to sugary foods and other empty-calorie snacks if she is allowed to consume them in unlimited amounts.

Your job is to draw the line and stick to it. Difficult yes—but certainly doable.

PORTION SIZE

Never serve an adult-size portion to your preschooler. This should be obvious, but often parents do just that. Interestingly, the Department of Pediatrics at the University of Colorado School of Medicine carried out a study involving a large group of parents and their preschool-age children and concluded that the amount of food served to the children was clearly related to the amounts the parents served themselves. So if you yourself have a huge appetite, beware! It may rub off and adversely affect your child. Remember: you can always give her a second helping if she is still hungry.

While on the subject of mealtime, here is another tip. Slow down the meal. In a study of four-year-olds, it was shown that a rapid eating style, characterized by increased mouthfuls of food per minute, may be a behavioral marker for the development of childhood obesity. A little conversation between courses, creating longer mealtimes, not only avoids these potentially harmful eating habits, but is also healthier for proper digestion. As mentioned in the section on family mealtime, our best advice is to eat family meals together at the table in a calm quiet environment.

Specific meal plans and appropriate snacks for your preschooler are included in Chapter 11, but in the meantime, here are 10 general guidelines to help you raise a healthy, happy, and normal weight preschooler:

1. Eat regular family meals together.

2. Limit portion sizes and eat slowly.

3. No soda or sugar-sweetened drinks.

4. Choose low-fat or skim milk.

5. "Fat-proof" the house (no junk foods available).

6. Make water the drink of choice.

7. Place your children on the "prudent" diet (outlined on page 123).

8. Decrease their amount of screen time to defeat their SOB syndrome.

9. Promote sufficient amounts of restful sleep.

10. Increase physical activity through fun, engaging, and active play.

Chapter 12
PHYSICAL ACTIVITIES FOR PRESCHOOLERS

I N A PREVIOUS BOOK, I referred to the time children spend in sedentary activities as "SOB syndrome" (Sitting On Butt Syndrome). Since that book was published over 40 years ago, SOB time has continued to increase. Besides television, we now have video games, computers, tablets, smart phones . . . the list of indoor distractions goes on. A 2015 survey of 350 families of children ages 6 months–4 years clearly indicates this. Conducted in an urban-income, minority population, the results showed that by age 4, half of the children had their own television sets and 75 percent of them had mobile devices, most often a tablet. There is now also less opportunity for outdoor physical activity due to safety issues and urban crowding. Even our preschoolers are now spending more of each day sitting in front of a screen, instead of spending time outdoors in physical activity.

No wonder so many kids are unfit, overweight, or obese.

In order to maintain normal weight and prevent childhood obesity, it is your job as a parent to find ways to reduce your child's SOB time. The Dietary Guidelines for Americans state that for children 2 years old and older, "Strong evidence supports that regular participation in physical activity helps maintain a healthy weight and prevents excess weight gain."

It does not take a genius to come to the same conclusion. But it *is* becoming more and more difficult for parents to ensure that their young children get enough physical exercise. Back in the "good old days" when I was young, before television and computers, when auto traffic and street crime were less of a threat, I would spend many hours outside each day with friends—running, jumping, playing games in the street, rolling around in the grass, and having a great time. Times have changed in a big way. Parents are now reluctant to allow their preschoolers out of doors without careful supervision. And given the realities of modern life, this is as it should be; the safety of your child should always come first.

But despite these sometimes difficult logistics, regular outdoor playtime is no less essential now than it was 40 years ago. It requires adequate and active supervision, certainly; rules must be established, and of course the play area or playground should be checked out to find and eliminate any safety hazards. Without exception, parents should make certain that their child always uses appropriate protective equipment, such as a bicycle helmet.

These difficulties in no way excuse the substitution of increased SOB time for outdoor activity and socialization. But now that many mothers are away at work during the day—another change from 40 years ago—they are not around to provide this necessary supervision. The result is that many preschoolers spend too much time indoors with a babysitter, watching hour upon hour of daytime TV. Others are in daycare or nursery school, with few opportunities for active, vigorous outdoor physical activity. (With this in mind, the Institute of Medicine recommends that child care facilities arrange for at least 15 minutes of physical activity each hour. We suggest you confirm that your child care center is following this recommendation. And while we're on this subject, we would advise that you also find out about the types of food and drinks they are feeding your child. According to the Centers for Disease Control and Prevention (CDC), many child care centers are now offering more healthful foods and more exercise, but it still is important to investigate the child care center your child attends.)

The results of increased S.O.B. time and decreased outdoor activity have been disastrous in terms of the obesity epidemic. Not to mention, the hazards of a sedentary lifestyle go way beyond obesity. It is considered a specific risk factor for future cardiovascular problems, such as heart attacks and hypertension.

A father of a 4-year-old once asked me, "You know, Andy is so laid back and calm that he can watch TV for three hours at a time without getting up even once. Isn't that great?" "No," I answered," it's not great at all. If he keeps it up, Andy will be on his way to real trouble." It took some time on my part to convince that father how important regular physical activity was for Andy's health and well-being. In this case, my efforts were successful. Andy is now playing No. 1 singles for his high school tennis team.

A large percentage of preschoolers are already TV and video game junkies. What this means is that, even when an opportunity for safe, supervised outdoor activity presents itself, it is hard to tear them away from their SOB time for a trip to the playground. Children who have been encouraged by their loving, well-meaning parents to "sit still and be good" and watch T.V. when they were toddlers are not very interested in active physical activity. They have learned to sit around and not get into trouble, rather than finding ways to run around and exercise.

These "old" habits (although not really old) are difficult to change. Instilling new physical activity habits for sedentary preschoolers requires active effort and involvement on your part. If you prefer to spend Sunday afternoons in front of the TV set (which I state at the risk of upsetting the football fans), it is less likely that you will interrupt your own SOB time to take your child outside to play.

Another important reason to encourage your preschooler to run, jump, and chase after thrown and kicked balls, unrelated to the prevention of obesity, is that regular exercise will make your child smarter. A correlation has been found between a child's aerobic fitness and his brain structure. The areas of the brain that are related to thinking and learning have been found to be larger among fit children as compared to unfit children.

A recent study conducted by researchers at the University of Illinois further confirms this correlation. A large group of young, school-aged children was divided, with half being placed on a wait list for afternoon physical activity programs, and the other half bused every day to the university, where they participated in fun-filled, structured physical activities for two hours. These activities included playing tag and kicking a soccer ball, exercises meant to improve both motor skills and endurance.

This was continued for a full school year. The results showed that the exercise group were fitter, had lost body fat, and displayed substantial improvement in their cognitive scores. Dr. Charles Hillman, who led this study, is quoted as follows: "Get your kids to be physically active for the sake of their brains and their health."

So, if your child is already a TV/video game junkie, what can you do to change things? During the preschool years, parental example is a mighty, potent force. This will change as your child gets older, and their peers and teachers begin to exert more influence, but for right now, it is *your* actions that are key to success or failure. By becoming more personally active, you will influence and shape her habits in positive ways. If you really get involved with your child, we are certain that she will quickly join in the fun, and will learn to enjoy vigorous physical activities. As an added bonus, you also will reap the health benefits of regular exercise.

If our goal is to be the prevention of childhood obesity, regular daily physical activity is necessary, regardless of whether your preschooler is normal weight or already overweight. Diet alone is not enough; free play must also be encouraged. The emphasis should be on having fun, exploring and experimenting (always under proper supervision).

Your youngster doesn't need acres of open spaces to get enough exercise. If you have no backyard of your own, I am sure there is a safe park or playground in your neighborhood. It would be great if you found one that has climbing equipment; if there are slides and swings, so much the better.

This reminds me of a call I got from the mother of 4-year-old Lucy: "Dr. Eden, we have to cancel Lucy's appointment. We were in the park and somebody stole my stroller with my purse in it. We are going to the police station to report the theft." When she came the next day, I asked her about her stolen purse and stroller. Neither had been found. I suggested that she not buy another stroller, point out that Lucy was perfectly capable of walking by herself, and that the exercise would be good for her, as Lucy was already a bit on the heavy side.

How much physical activity does your preschooler need each day to become fit and strong? How much outdoor activity is needed to prevent her from becoming overweight or obese? The easy answer is, the more the better. Another answer comes from the most recent Institute of Medicine report, "Early Obesity Prevention Policies," that states that preschoolers require at least 3 hours of physical activity per day. We encourage at least 1 hour of such activity per day be moderate to vigorous structured active play. This vigorous physical activity should be outdoors, if possible. Research and common sense both tell us that children are more active outdoors than indoors. Going outside to play also cuts down on accidental damage to family members, furniture, and any valuable vases you might have to hand.

Allow us to briefly discuss the two types of physical activity, namely unstructured and structured. Your child should be involved in both types each day. The following are some examples of each:

Unstructured

1. Playing on or around outdoor playground structures (swings, slides, etc.)

2. Riding tricycles, scooters and riding toys

3. Digging and building in a sandbox

4. Running after a ball

5. Hitting and catching balls

Structured

1. Setting up an obstacle course

2. Aiming and throwing a ball into bucket or hoop

3. Dancing to music and learning certain movements

4. Playing "Simple Simon"

This is a good time to discuss physical activity and calories. Calories are defined as the energy contained within foods. When you eat, you take in calories; when you exercise, you burn calories. Both diet and exercise are, at some level, about the calories in versus the calories out. The number to remember is that one pound of fat equals 3,500 calories. By burning up 3,500 calories, you lose 1 pound of fat. There are seven days in a week, so if you lose 500 calories a day, it translates to 3,500 calories per week, which equals a 1 pound of weight loss. That's all you need to know to do the job.

The following is a table that will give you some ideas about how physical activity affects weight loss. Don't worry: your preschooler is competent enough to easily handle all these physical activities, and more.

CALORIE-BURNING ACTIVITIES

Exercise	30 Minutes	Weight Loss/ Month
Brisk Walk	175 Calories	1½ pounds
Jogging	225	2 pounds
Running	450	3½ pounds
Swimming	340	3 pounds
Biking	250	2 pounds
Sweeping Floor	75	¾ pound

This table illustrates that daily active physical activity is necessary to maintain normal weight. Without daily calorie burning activities, your preschooler will slowly but surely put on extra pounds of fat, even if eating a normal diet.

As we pointed out earlier, the prevention of childhood obesity does not require a preschooler to lose weight (with the possible exception being markedly obese children). In such cases, your physician may advise a weight reduction program, but never more than 1 pound per month.

In discussing the promotion of active physical activity for children, a question that always comes up is, "What age should a child start playing organized sports or go to a gym?" There are many preschool programs in schools and communities across the country; this has become big business for gyms and workout centers. One such program, CrossFit Kids, has 700 classes in the United States for children ages 3–5 years. We certainly do not believe that such structured programs at this early age are necessary in order to raise a healthy and fit preschooler. However, if these classes are short (lasting 30 minutes or less), are relaxed and fun-filled and you can afford the expense, go ahead. We *do* advise checking out the program first and making certain that it fits these criteria.

The following are some specific suggestions to help your preschooler develop a love for vigorous physical activity, which will in turn give her strength, agility, stamina, coordination, in addition to protecting her from becoming overweight or obese:

Swimming: Freestyle water play (with plenty of splashing) is a terrific activity you can share with your child. Of course, never allow him in the water alone and unsupervised. Swimming is one of the "carry-over" sports that a person can continue throughout life, and so should be encouraged. It is never too early for swimming lessons, especially if your local YMCA or health club offers beginner classes. With proper instruction, he can learn basic swimming skills and techniques, along with water safety rules.

Dance classes: Well-suited for both for girls and boys, lessons in modern jazz, tap, and ballet can be started during the preschool years. Dancing provides opportunities not only for physical exercise, but also for developing rhythm, coordination, discipline and socialization skills.

Family outings: It may be hard to find the time, but family outings together spent hiking, motivation climbing (hill climbing), apple picking, or just taking a long walk to a particular destination are well within the capabilities of preschoolers. In fact, you'll probably tire out before your child! These outings become indelibly imprinted into your preschooler's happy memory bank.

Roughhousing: There is nothing like a gentle wrestling match with your preschooler so they can experience not only vigorous exercise, but also hugs, kisses, and laughter, all of which are important for the emotional well-being of everyone involved. You can do it on the bed or on the floor (with a rug or mat) anytime you have a few minutes. Note: one exception is before bedtime, when vigorous physical activity and excitement can disrupt proper sleep. We are strong advocates of this form of physical activity. It uses all her muscles, increases both strength and flexibility, and brings you together in a unique and wonderful way. *Both my children, now grown up with children of their own, remind me that our wrestling matches on their beds are one of their most pleasant childhood memories.*

Anti-SOB activities: This refers to anything that discourages SOB syndrome and gets her moving instead of sitting, in order to burn up calories. It includes walking instead of driving; letting her walk instead of pushing her on a stroller is another strategy. It also includes getting her to help with household chores like sweeping the floor, making her bed, and taking out the garbage (it's never too early to put your child to work).

Scooters, tricycles, and riding toys: This should always be an outdoor activity. All preschoolers love to ride around as part of imaginary play. They develop agility, balance. and leg strength. Remember to practice sun safety—the use of appropriate sunscreen when your preschooler is playing outside is very important. Some parents only think of sunscreen when at the beach; don't forget, the sun shines just as brightly everywhere.

Athletics: This is a tricky subject during these preschool years. Many parents are already looking forward to raising the next Derek Jeter or Roger Federer, or an Olympic gold medal gymnast. I have no problem with these expectations, but I do take exception with parents pushing their children too hard and too fast at this young age. Most authorities believe that intensive training in any sport should not begin until the child is at least 6 years old. I personally think that it should start later than that, at around 7 or 8. Yes, I know about Andre Agassi hitting a tennis ball over and over when he was 3 or 4 years old. But if you read his book, you'll note that he hated every minute of it. There are a number of sports and physical activities that are appropriate for a 3–5 year old, including soccer, running, jumping, and learning to throw and catch a ball—so long as you don't take any of it *too* seriously. There will be plenty of time later on to develop particular skills in a specific sport. The idea now is to help your child build up the strength, coordination, speed, and stamina that are necessary to excel in any sport.

In summary, there are five important obesity prevention guidelines related to exercise:

1. Encourage at least 3 hours of physical activity each day, one of which should be structured and vigorous.

2. Fight the SOB syndrome.

3. Encourage outdoor physical activity each day.

4. Limit TV and screen time to one hour per day.

5. Encourage development of basic motor skills such as running, swimming, jumping, throwing and catching a ball.

Not only is regular physical activity beneficial in preventing childhood obesity, but it is also important psychologically, helping to increase self-esteem and self-confidence while decreasing anxiety and depression. The guidelines and recommendations about nutrition and physical activity that we have discussed are appropriate for all toddlers and preschoolers, whether they are normal weight, overweight, or obese.

The prevention of childhood obesity is relatively easy for many, and while with some 3–5-year-olds it can be quite difficult, it *can* be done. Careful monitoring of your child's BMI percentile is absolutely essential to ensure success. Preschoolers who are at greatest risk for obesity later on in life include those who have reached a BMI at or greater than the 85th percentile. Those who have a rapid weight gain resulting in the upward crossing of percentiles toward the 85th are also in danger. If your preschooler fits these "high-risk" categories you must discuss it with her physician. It is obvious that changes either in her diet, her physical activity, or both are required. As stated at the start of this book, the treatment of obesity in the older child is usually unsuccessful.

Prevention is the best solution.

PART III

MEAL PLANS FOR TODDLERS AND PRESCHOOLERS

TODDLER MEAL PLAN (AGES 1–3 YEARS)

THE FOLLOWING MENU, INCLUDING MEALS and snacks, is designed for healthy toddlers without dietary restrictions and is based on an average of 1,000–1,200 calories per day. Toddlers have little tummies, so offer two to three daily snacks spaced at least two hours apart from mealtime. Serve milk or water with meals and snacks. Two cups of milk every day (or dairy equivalents) will provide most of the calcium your toddler needs for bone growth without interfering with their appetite for other foods. For toddlers less than 2 years old, offer whole milk. If your toddler is overweight or you have a family history of obesity, heart disease, or high cholesterol, your pediatrician may recommend reduced-fat milk (2 percent). For toddlers ages 2–3 years, serve skim milk or low-fat milk (1 percent).

If your toddler is 1 year old and rejecting cow milk, try mixing it with familiar formula or breast milk to gradually gain acceptance. Adjust the mixture over time until it becomes 100 percent cow's milk. You can also explore other sources of calcium such as calcium-fortified soy beverages or almond milk, fortified breads and cereals, cooked dried beans, and dark green vegetables like broccoli, bok choy, and kale.

WEEKLY MENU

Sunday

BREAKFAST

Nutrient-Loaded Oatmeal (1 bowl)

LUNCH

Easy Microwave Spiced Cod
Cauliflower snowballs (¼ cup)
Cheese sauce, (2 tablespoons, optional)

DINNER

Veggie Spaghetti Squash
Unsweetened applesauce (½ cup)

Monday

BREAKFAST

Waffle Strips with Banana Blackberry Dip

LUNCH

Cheese muffin with ¼ cup creamed spinach

DINNER

Alphabet Tomato Soup (1 cup)

Tuesday

BREAKFAST

Little Bear's Breakfast Porridge

LUNCH

Avocado Greek Yogurt with Crunchy Dippers

DINNER

Panko-Crusted Tilapia Bites
Apple Mango Dip

Wednesday

BREAKFAST

Green Eggs and Ham

LUNCH

California Rotini with Cheese or Marinara Sauce

DINNER

Protein-Packed Brown Rice Bowl

Thursday

BREAKFAST

Soy Good Sunshine Smoothie

LUNCH

Nut Butter Smiley Face
Diced fruit (¼ cup)

DINNER

Hummus Chip Chicken Bites
Fruit-Spiked Sweet Potatoes

Friday

BREAKFAST

French Toast and Peaches

LUNCH

Bulgur Pilaf
½ a serving of string cheese
Diced fruit (¼ cup)

DINNER

Beef and Bean Jack-O'-Lantern

Saturday

BREAKFAST

Early Bird Yogurt Parfait

LUNCH

Tuna Melt Triangles

DINNER

Cinnamon Stew

Nutrient-Loaded Oatmeal

Active time: 5 minutes
Cook time: 1 minute
Serves: 1

½ cup water, skim, or 1 percent milk*
¼ ripe banana, mashed
½ tablespoon almond butter
¼ cup dry Quaker 1-minute oats
¼ cup water
Dash of cinnamon
* For ages 1–2 years, use whole milk dairy.

➤ Boil water or milk. In a small bowl, stir banana with almond butter and add dry oats. Gradually stir in liquid until thickened to desired consistency. Sprinkle with cinnamon.

Waffle Strips with Banana Blackberry Dip

Active time: 5 minutes
Cook time: 5 minutes
Serves: 1

¼ cup blackberries, fresh or thawed from frozen package
1 tablespoon water
½ small banana, sliced
1 whole grain frozen waffle, or 4 mini waffles
Blender

➤ Place the blackberries in a saucepan with water and cook for about 2 minutes. You will see the fruit juices start to ooze out of the berries. Blend the cooked blackberries and banana until smooth.

Prepare waffle according to package directions, and cut into bite-size strips (a pizza slicer creates instant waffle strips). Serve with banana blackberry dip.

Alternatively, you can spoon the dip directly onto the waffle, fold it over, and enjoy as a fruit sandwich. Feel free to create your own berry combination using raspberries and blueberries.

Little Bear's Breakfast Porridge

Active time: **5 minutes**
Cook time: **20 minutes**
Serves: 6

2 cups 1 percent milk*
1 cup water
1 cup uncooked amaranth
1 small apple, peeled and chopped
1 tablespoon water
1 small pear, peeled and chopped
Pinch of cinnamon or nutmeg (optional)
* For ages 1–2 years, use whole milk.

➤ Bring water, milk and amaranth to a boil in a medium saucepan. Simmer and cook covered for 20 minutes (stirring occasionally) until the mixture becomes thick, resembling porridge.

While the amaranth is cooking, place the chopped apple in a saucepan and add the 1 tablespoon water. Cover and cook over low heat for 4 minutes. Add the chopped pear and cook with apple until tender, an additional 4–5 minutes.

Stir in the stewed fruit and divide porridge between 6 serving bowls. Sprinkle with cinnamon or nutmeg.

Make more to store: Save time by preparing a batch of whole grains. Cooked grains will keep in in the fridge for 3–4 days. Just add a little water or milk and reheat. The amaranth will soak up most of the liquid in this porridge. For a plain amaranth dish, boil 6 cups liquid to 1 cup amaranth, drain the cooked grain through a fine mesh strainer, and enjoy!

Amaranth is a tiny seed with super grain qualities—it's gluten-free and contains all nine essential amino acids, making it a complete protein. Amaranth is also a star source of iron, magnesium, and phosphorous. Inspired by a classic childhood storybook, your toddler will love this golden, nutty grain recipe when cooked to a porridge-like consistency. Millet, a light yellow whole grain, milder in flavor, also works well as a hot cereal. Millet has a soft, fluffy texture, tastes similar to cornmeal and is brimming with fiber and B vitamins.

Green Eggs and Ham

Active time: **5 minutes**
Cook time: **5 minutes**
Serves: **2**

2 large eggs
¼ cup 1 percent milk*
2 tablespoons crumbled feta cheese
1 slice of lower-sodium deli ham, diced
1 teaspoon extra-virgin olive oil
1 cup pre-washed baby arugula and spinach, torn into pieces
2 mini whole grain pitas (1-ounce each), sliced into triangles
* For ages 1–2 years, use whole milk.

➤ In a mixing bowl, beat the eggs. Stir in milk, cheese, and ham, blending well.

Swirl oil in nonstick skillet over medium heat. Sauté arugula and spinach until leaves start to wilt. Add egg mixture to skillet and cook over low, stirring frequently, until eggs are cooked through, about 2 minutes. Divide between two bowls and serve with pita triangles.

Depending on your toddler's preference, this recipe works great with miniature utensils or as a first finger-food sandwich.

Soy Good Sunshine Smoothie

Active time: **5 minutes**
Cook time: **None**
Serves: **2**

1 cup light vanilla soy milk
3 ounces silken tofu
1 tablespoon ground flaxseed meal
1 tablespoon smooth almond butter
⅓ cup canned yams in light syrup*
4–6 ice cubes
*You can substitute ¾ cup sliced frozen peaches for the yams.

➤ Place all ingredients in blender, cover, and whip until smooth.

Tofu is made from the curds of soybeans, in much the same way cheese is made from milk. Tofu acts like a sponge and will absorb the flavor of its neighboring ingredients. You can use firm tofu in a stir-fry, soft tofu in creamy dips, and silken tofu in smoothies as a plant source of protein. and calcium.

French Toast and Peaches

Active time: **5 minutes**
Cook time: **5 minutes**
Serves: **2**

1 egg
¼ cup milk*
1 teaspoon vanilla extract
2 slices whole grain bread
1 teaspoon of soft margarine, made with vegetable oil
½ cup diced peaches, fresh or canned, in water or juice
2 tablespoons vanilla yogurt, divided*
* For ages 1–2 years, use whole milk, dairy

➤ Scramble egg with milk and vanilla extract. Dip bread slices into egg mixture, turning gently to coat both sides. Heat a nonstick skillet over medium-high heat. Melt margarine in pan. Add coated bread slices; cook 2 minutes on each side until lightly browned. Slice French toast into sticks or bite-size squares. Serve with diced peaches and a dollop of yogurt.

Early Bird Yogurt Parfait

Active time: **5 minutes**
Cook time: **None**
Serves: 1

½ cup Greek yogurt, any flavor*
¼ cup diced fruit, fresh or canned in water or juice
½ cup low-sugar whole grain cereal
* For ages 1–2 years, use whole milk dairy

➤ In a small bowl or clear plastic cup, spoon a layer of yogurt, top with fruit, sprinkle cereal, and repeat process to create a parfait.

Select whole grain cereals with less than 5 grams of sugar such as Cascadian Farms Purely O's, General Mills Cheerios, General Mills Kix, or Kashi® Heart to Heart® Honey Toasted Oat Cereal.

This instant breakfast is just what your toddler needs for a nutritious start to a busy day—packed with an energy trio of whole grains, fruit, and high-protein Greek yogurt.

Easy Microwave Spiced Cod

Active time: **2 minutes**
Cook time: **3–4 minutes**
Serves: **6**

6-ounce cod fillet, skin removed
¼ cup unsalted vegetable broth or stock*
1 teaspoon soft margarine or extra-virgin olive oil
Seasoning: dash of dried dill + garlic powder or Chinese 5 Spice
     Powder (⅛ teaspoon)
* When buying cartons or cans at the store, note that some stock
     might have a slightly deeper flavor and lower sodium than
     others, depending on the manufacturer.

➤ Pour broth in a microwave-safe dish and place fish inside. Dab fish
with margarine or oil. Sprinkle with seasoning, cover with plastic
wrap, and poke a few small holes in the wrap to allow venting.
Microwave on high for 3–4 minutes, or until fish flakes easily with a
fork. Cooking time may vary slightly depending on your oven. Flake
the fish into bite-size pieces and mix with cheese sauce.

*Amp up the flavor of traditional dishes with Chinese five spice
powder. This pantry staple is like a spice rack in a bottle. The
blend contains cinnamon, star anise, fennel, ground cloves, and
black pepper, which adds a delicate balance of sweet and spicy
flavors to any meal. Not only are you slashing sodium and sugar,
but you are loading up on antioxidants.*

Cauliflower Snowballs

Active time: **10 minutes**
Cook time: **5–10 minutes**
Serves: **6**

1 small head cauliflower or 2 cups frozen cauliflower florets
1 cup unsalted vegetable broth or stock*
½ cup skim milk or skim plus milk (skim plus has a creamier
    consistency)
1 tablespoon grated parmesan cheese

➤ *When buying cartons or cans at the store, some stock might have a slightly deeper flavor and less sodium than others, depending on the manufacturer.

If using frozen cauliflower, steam in microwave according to package directions.

If using fresh cauliflower: Pull off the outer leaves and cut off stem. Using a paring knife in a circular motion, cut around the core and voila! The florets will easily pull apart. Rinse florets in colander. In a medium saucepan, boil broth. Place 2 cups of cauliflower in steam basket and refrigerate the rest. Cover and steam for 8–10 minutes until florets can easily be pierced with a fork. Make sure the steam basket is close to the broth but not touching it.

Place cooked florets in a mixing bowl and mash with a fork while slowly blending in milk and cheese. Stir in the flaked fish. You can also use a handheld electric mixer or immersion blender for a creamier consistency. With an ice-cream scoop, stack 2 cauliflower snow balls in a bowl, and serve.

Make colored snowballs by using purple and orange cauliflower varieties, too! Double the recipe and freeze leftovers. You can also finely chop or grate leftover cauliflower florets for a tasty nutrient-packed pizza topping.

Cheese Muffin

Active time: **5 minutes**
Cook time: **None**
Serves: **2**

1 whole grain English muffin, sliced in half or 2 Vitatop muffins
¼ ripe avocado, mashed
1 slice reduced-fat cheddar cheese*
* For ages 1–2 years, use whole milk yogurt and cheese.

➤ Lightly toast English muffin halves. If using Vitatops, defrost according to package instructions. Spread 2 tablespoons of avocado on each Vitatop or English Muffin half, add cheese and close up sandwich. Microwave muffin for 10 seconds until cheese is melted. Cut into bite-size pieces. Serve with creamed spinach dip.

Vitatops are whole grain muffin tops that come in assorted flavors made without artificial preservatives or additives. They can be found in the frozen section of your grocery store or available at www.vitalicious.com.

Creamed Spinach

Active time: **5 minutes**
Cook time: **3 minutes**
Serves: **2**

3 cups fresh or pre-washed baby spinach leaves
2 tablespoons nonfat Greek yogurt*
¼ cup reduced-fat mozzarella cheese*
Pinch of nutmeg (optional)
* For ages 1–2 years, use whole milk yogurt and cheese.

➤ Arrange spinach in a microwave-safe dish, loosely covered, and cook
for 3 minutes until leaves are wilted. Let cool slightly, and chop spinach leaves. Stir in Greek yogurt and cheese until smooth. Add a dash
of nutmeg.

*Baby spinach is an ideal leafy green for toddlers—the leaves are
smaller, more tender, and delicate than full-size spinach. Greens
shrink when cooked, so buy plenty! Refrigerate in a plastic bag
up to 5 days.*

California Rotini with Cheese or Marinara Sauce

Active time: **5 minutes**
Cook time: **10 minutes**
Serves: **2**

1 cup cooked tri-color rotini pasta (measure ⅔ cup dry pasta)
1 cup California blend vegetables (broccoli, cauliflower, carrots),
　　from frozen package
¼ cup reduced-sodium vegetable broth (optional)

➤ Cook pasta according to package directions. Steam vegetables in microwave according to package instructions. Cut into bite-size pieces or puree with broth to desired consistency. Drizzle with cheese sauce.

> *You can boil a batch of pasta and refrigerate leftovers for 3–5 days. When fresh-picked vegetables are frozen, nutrients are locked in, making them a healthy shortcut to an instant vitamin-boosted dish for your toddler.*

Cheese Sauce

Active time: **5 minutes**
Cook time: **5–6 minutes**
Serves: **6**

1 tablespoon butter or margarine made with vegetable oil
1 tablespoon all-purpose flour
1 cup 1 percent milk or soymilk*
⅓ cup reduced-fat grated cheese
* For ages 1–2 years, use whole milk yogurt and cheese

➤ Melt butter or margarine in a saucepan over low heat. Add flour and stir with a whisk to make a smooth paste, about 1–2 minutes. Slowly add milk, bring to a boil and simmer on low heat for an additional 3–4 minutes, stirring until sauce has thickened. Stir in the grated cheese until melted. Spoon sauce over pasta. Alternatively, top pasta with 2 tablespoons of store bought marinara sauce.

Makes ¾ cup sauce (use 2 tablespoons per portion). Refrigerate leftover sauce for 3–4 days in a sealed container or freeze 4–6 months.

Nut Butter Smiley Face

Active time: **5 minutes**
Cook time: **None**
Serves: **2**

2 slices of white whole wheat or whole wheat bread
2 tablespoons smooth peanut butter, almond butter, or sunflower
    butter, divided
½ banana, sliced into 6 thin circles
2 teaspoons all-fruit strawberry or grape preserves
¼ peeled apple, chopped into tiny squares
Small juice glass

➤ Punch out a circle in the center of each slice of bread using the bottom
of a small drinking glass. Reserve two crusts. Spread each circle with
1 tablespoon of nut butter and stick on the bananas to create "eyes"
and a "nose." Using a butter knife, swirl a smiley face with the fruit
preserves and place the bread crust on top to create a mouth. Press in
the apple squares as teeth.

Choose natural nut butters such as Smucker's or Barney Butter. Some natural food stores serve pure nut butters churned fresh from a machine with no additives. Refrigerate opened containers upside down to keep the nut butter smooth and prolong shelf life.

Both white whole wheat bread and regular whole wheat bread are made with whole grains but differ in the types of wheat used. White whole wheat bread is made from white wheat, which lacks bran color. It also has a milder flavor and softer texture, which may be more appealing to toddlers who reject regular whole wheat. Regular whole wheat bread is made from red wheat, which is darker in color and has a coarser texture.

White bread is made with refined grains, which go through a process that strips out essential layers of the grain—along with some of the nutrients and fiber. Some of the vitamins and minerals in refined grains are added back through "enrichment" but your best bet is to choose breads that say "100 percent whole grain" or list "whole wheat" as the first ingredient. A label may simply say "white wheat," which is not as nutritious as "white whole wheat."

Avocado Greek Yogurt

Active time: **5 minutes**
Cook time: **None**
Serves: **2**

Yogurt:
½ ripe avocado
2 tablespoons nonfat vanilla Greek yogurt*
2 tablespoons mashed, ripe berries or bananas (optional)

Crunchy Dippers:
½ cup: cucumber, grape tomatoes, and carrots, cut into bite-size
    pieces
½ whole grain English muffin or pita, toasted and sliced into
    squares.
* For 1–2 years olds, use whole milk yogurt.

➤ Slice open avocado and remove inner pit. Wrap and store half the avocado in refrigerator for future use. Spoon the flesh out of remaining half of avocado and mash with fork. Stir in yogurt and fruit if desired. Divide yogurt between two bowls and serve each portion with ¼ cup vegetables and two toasted whole grain squares.

> *Squeezing a little lemon or lime juice on avocado flesh before wrapping will prevent browning in the refrigerator.*

Bulgur Pilaf

Active time: **10 minutes**
Cook time: **15 minutes**
Serves: 6

1 tablespoon extra-virgin olive oil
1 cup chopped onions, fresh or frozen
1 cup chopped mixed bell peppers, fresh or frozen
1 garlic clove, minced
1 cup uncooked bulgur
2 cups unsalted vegetable broth or stock

➤ Heat oil in saucepan over medium heat and sauté onion, peppers, and garlic until softened, about 4–5 minutes. Add bulgur, coating the grains in oil. Add broth and simmer for 10–12 minutes until all the liquid is absorbed.

> *Bulgur is cracked wheat that has been parboiled, dried, and broken into granules, making it a nutritious fast food for those new to whole grain cooking. Bulgur has more fiber than quinoa, oats, millet, buckwheat, or corn. Sometimes referred to as "Middle Eastern pasta," bulgur is a star source of protein, magnesium, and phosphorous.*

Tuna Melt Triangles

Active time: **10 minutes**
Cook time: **5 minutes**
Serves: **6**

1 hard-boiled egg, mashed
¼ cup low-fat plain yogurt**
2 tablespoons mayonnaise made with olive or canola oil
6-ounce can light tuna packed in water, drained and flaked
3 (6-inch) whole grain tortillas or flatbreads such as *Flatouts**
3 slices of light Swiss cheese*
*Flatouts are available a grocery stores or can be ordered at
   www.flatoutbread.com.
** For ages 1–2 years, use whole milk dairy.

➤ To hard-boil the egg, put the egg in a saucepan, and then add enough
cold water to cover it by ½ inch. Bring water to a boil over high heat.
Remove from burner and cover pan. Let eggs stand in hot water,
about 12 minutes. Run cold water into pot to stop cooking. Gently
peel egg.
   Preheat oven to 350°F. In a mixing bowl, combine yogurt and
mayonnaise. Stir in tuna and egg. Divide tuna mixture and spread
evenly over each tortilla or flatbread; top with cheese and fold in
half. Bake in oven until cheese is melted. Slice tuna melts into bite-size
triangles.

*Make more to store: Boil a batch of eggs, and refrigerate them
shell-on for up to 1 week.*

Veggie Spaghetti Squash

Active time: **15 minutes**
Cook time: **30*–80 minutes**
Serves: **8–12**

1 whole spaghetti squash
Topping, per single portion:
1 tablespoon tomato sauce
1–2 tablespoons shredded mozzarella cheese
1 tablespoon vegetable broth (if using as a puree)

➤ Preheat oven to 375°F. Rinse squash and poke holes around the entire surface using a small sharp knife. Place squash on a foil lined sheet and bake in oven for 40 minutes per side, turning halfway through cooking time. Remove and let cool. Slice squash in half lengthwise. With a spoon, scoop out the seeds and discard. Using a fork, scrape out the inner spaghetti squash strands.

   *Quick microwave method: Pierce squash all over with a small sharp knife. Place in a microwave-safe bowl covered with a damp paper towel; cook on high for 5 minutes, turn the squash, and repeat process 2–3 times until squash is tender, approximately 20 minutes (when a knife slides in pretty easily, the squash is done). Let cool. Slice squash in half lengthwise, scoop out inner seeds, and remove spaghetti strands.

   Divide squash into ½-cup portions and top with tomato sauce and cheese. Refrigerate cooked squash for up to 3 days or freeze for future use.

   For pureed version: Blend squash with broth and tomato sauce. Sprinkle with cheese. You can also puree the squash with cinnamon and unsweetened applesauce.

> *Winter squashes can be substituted for one another in recipes and these include acorn, butternut, delicata, Hubbard, pumpkin, and spaghetti. Peaks in late fall through winter.*

Alphabet Tomato Soup

Active time: **5 minutes**
Cook time: **10 minutes**
Serves: **2**

½ cup (2 ounces) dry whole grain alphabet pasta* or other
   small-shaped pasta such as ditalini or pastina* (about 2
   ounces dry)
1 cup frozen chopped broccoli
14.5-ounce can reduced-sodium tomato soup such as Amy's
   Organic Chunky Tomato Bisque
⅓ cup cannellini beans, rinsed and drained
Optional garnish: 1 tablespoon finely crushed pine nuts or grated
   parmesan cheese.
*2 ounces dry pasta measures ⅓ to ½ cup depending on the
   shape.

➤ Prepare alphabet pasta according to package directions and add
broccoli during the last 3–4 minutes of cooking time. Drain in small
colander and set aside. In a large pot over medium-high heat, stir
the tomato soup with the beans. When soup is hot, add pasta with
broccoli and simmer for 1–2 minutes. Sprinkle nuts or cheese. Puree
soup in blender if desired. Let cool slightly and serve warm.

*Select pasta with the word "whole durum wheat" listed as the
first ingredient such as Eden Organic Vegetable Alphabets or
Barilla Whole Grain Shapes available at grocery stores or online
at www.amazon.com.*

Panko-Crusted Tilapia Bites with Apple Mango Dip

Active time: **20 minutes**
Cook time: **20–30 minutes**
Serves: **4–6**

Panko-Crusted Tilapia Bites:
8 ounces tilapia or other white flesh fish fillet such as flounder, sole or cod
1 tablespoon mayonnaise made with olive or canola oil
½ cup panko (Japanese breadcrumbs)
Dash of seasoning: garlic and onion powder
Cooking spray or vegetable oil

Apple Mango Dip
1 apple, peeled, cored, and chopped
1 tablespoon water
½ cup chopped mango, fresh or thawed from frozen package
Blender

➤ *Panko-Crusted Tilapia Bites*
Preheat oven to 425°F. Spread mayonnaise on both sides of fish fillet and gently slice into 4 strips. Combine breadcrumbs with seasoning. In a zip top bag, combine fish strips with breadcrumb mixture and shake until coated. Place fish in a baking dish lightly coated with oil or spray, and bake uncovered until fish flakes easily with a fork, 15–20 minutes.

➤ *Apple Mango Dip*
Place the chopped apple in a saucepan and add the water. Cover and cook over low heat for 6–8 minutes, until tender. Blend cooked apple with mango until smooth. Drizzle over fish sticks or serve as a dip. Alternatively, you can substitute the mango with canned pineapple packed in water or juice.

Pairing fruit with fish introduces toddlers to a unique flavor combination. For a family recipe, you can whip up a tropical salsa using diced apples, mangoes, chopped cilantro, and a squeeze of lime juice.

The mango is a symbol of love in India and a basket of mangoes is considered a gesture of friendship. In many Latin American countries, mango on a stick with the skin peeled back is sold by street vendors.

Protein-Packed Brown Rice Bowl

Active time: **10 minutes**
Cook time: **10 minutes**
Serves: **4**

½ cup cooked peas from frozen package
1 cup of cooked instant rice such as Uncle Ben's 90-second
    Ready Rice
1 frozen veggie burger or ½ cup soft tofu (about 4 ounces, patted
    dry with paper towels)
¼ cup reduced-fat shredded cheddar cheese*
1 cup tomato sauce
* For 1–2 years olds, use whole milk cheese.

➤ Cook peas and brown rice according to package directions. If using
tofu, mash with fork; if using veggie burger, prepare according to
package directions and crumble into small pieces.

    In a large skillet, heat the tomato sauce. Mix in peas, rice, and
crumbled veggie burger. Stir in cheese until melted through. Divide
mixture into toddler-size bowls.

---

*Select a veggie burger made with whole grains with at least 10
grams of protein such as Dr. Praeger's Black Bean Burger or
Amy's Organic Light in Sodium California Veggie Burger.*

Hummus Chip Chicken Bites

Active time: 15 minutes
Cook time: 30 minutes
Serves: 4–6

Cooking spray
1 ounce sweet potato chips, (about 10–15 chips)*
8 ounces boneless, skinless chicken breasts, cut into strips
½ cup hummus, divided
Drizzle of peanut or canola oil

➤ Preheat oven to 400°F and coat a baking sheet with cooking spray. Crush chips in a zip-top bag. Spread chicken strips with a thin layer of hummus (about 1 tablespoon per strip) and place in zip-top bag, coating with crushed chips. Arrange chicken on baking sheet in a single layer, lightly drizzle with oil, and cook 10–15 minutes per side, until golden brown. Let cool and cut into bite-size pieces.

* *Sweet potato chips add a delightful crunch and a hefty dose of vitamin A that your toddler will gobble up. For a colorful mix, try Terra Exotic Vegetable Chips made with parsnip, taro, sweet potato, yucca, and batata.*

Fruit-Spiked Sweet Potatoes

Active time: 5 minutes
Cook time: 8 minutes
Serves: 4–6

1 sweet potato
½ cup canned fruit, packed in water or 100 percent juice
   (pineapple or orange segments) diced or pureed in a blender.

➤ Using a fork, prick holes on all sides of potato, and place in a micro-wave-safe bowl with plastic wrap. Poke a small hole in the wrap leaving an air vent. Cook on high for 8 minutes, turning halfway through cooking time. Slice open and let cool. Scoop out the potato flesh into a mixing bowl and combine with fruit.

The natural sweetness of sweet potato blended with fruit makes this an all year round favorite.

Beef and Bean Jack-O'-Lantern

Active time: **5 minutes**
Cook time: **10 minutes**
Serves: **4**

Cooking spray
4 ounces 90 percent lean ground beef
2 tablespoons tomato sauce
½ cup vegetarian refried beans
½ cup Monterey Jack cheese, divided
4 whole grain tortillas

➤ Preheat oven to 350°F and coat a baking sheet with cooking spray. Heat a nonstick skillet over medium heat and cook beef until browned about 5–6 minutes. Swirl in the tomato sauce with beans and simmer until heated through, about 2 minutes. Divide the beef mixture between two tortillas, leaving a ½ inch border around the edge; cover with a layer of grated cheese. Using a knife, cut two triangles for eyes and a crescent for a mouth on the other two tortillas. Lay the completed jack-o'-lantern faces on top of each filled tortilla.

Arrange quesadillas on baking sheet. Cook in oven for 3–5 minutes until the cheese melts. Divide each quesadilla into six bite sized wedges.

Canned pinto beans provide the base for a healthy meal without the fuss. Try Amy's Light in Sodium Organic Vegetarian refried beans that contain a goodie bag of nutrients, including dietary fiber, protein, and iron.

Cinnamon Stew

Active time: **20 minutes**
Cook time: **20 minutes**
Serves: 8

1 tablespoon extra-virgin olive oil
8 ounces boneless, skinless chicken breast, cut into small cubes
1 sweet potato, peeled, and chopped
1 apple, peeled, cored, and chopped
2 cups reduced-sodium chicken stock or broth
⅛–¼ teaspoon ground cinnamon
2 cups cooked brown rice or small-shaped pasta such as pastina
    or ditalini
3 tablespoons reduced-fat shredded Swiss or mozzarella cheese,
    divided (optional)*
* For 1–2 years olds, use whole milk cheese.

➤ Organic, whole grain (toddler-size) pastas such as Eden Organic
Kamut Ditalini and Eden Organic Vegetable Alphabets are available
at www.edenfoods.com

In a saucepan, heat the oil. Add the chicken cubes, and sauté
for 6–8 minutes, until no longer pink. Add the sweet potato, apple,
and cinnamon and pour in the stock. Bring to a boil, then cover and
simmer for 15 minutes. Stir the stew a few times. Remove from heat
and let cool. Prepare the grain according to package instructions.

Divide stew into individual portions. Alternatively, blend to
a puree for a smoother consistency. Top each portion with ¼ cup
cooked grain and sprinkle with cheese, if desired.

Make more to store: This recipe is suitable for freezing leftovers.
Simply thaw and reheat for an instant nutritious meal. You can substitute chicken with 90 percent lean ground beef or turkey.

*Once used in love potions and traditional medicines, cinnamon
is a sweet spice that is so versatile—it goes well in savory dishes
like soups and stews, and can do wonders on meat and chicken.
Cinnamon is oatmeal's best friend at breakfast and adds a tasty
accent to fruit-based desserts.*

A healthy snack portion is based on a 4-ounce bowl or plastic food container, unless otherwise specified. Snacks marked with an * are accompanied with a recipe. For dairy snacks, offer whole milk products to toddlers under 2 years old. For toddlers ages 2–3 years, select reduced-fat yogurt and cheeses, skim, 1 percent, soy or unsweetened non-dairy milks.

Fill a Snack Bowl with . . .

1. "ABC" yogurt: Combine ¼ mashed avocado, 2 tablespoons mashed banana, 2 tablespoons cherry yogurt.

2. Five frozen yogurt drops: Fill a plastic zip-top bag with flavored yogurt, snip off one of the corners and squeeze drops of yogurt on a paper plate. Freeze the drops until solid (about 2 hours) and serve. Store leftovers in a freezer-proof container.

3. Roasted Veggie Chips* and dip: Fill half a snack bowl with Roasted Veggie Chips and serve with 1 tablespoon hummus or marinara sauce for dipping. Alternatively, steam ¼ cup frozen chopped broccoli, cauliflower, or carrots in microwave-safe dish and serve with dip.

4. Pear and cheese: Slice one quarter of a pear into bite-size pieces and thinly spread (or dip) with 1 tablespoon ricotta, brie, or goat cheese.

5. Quick chili parfait: 1–2 tablespoons canned chili, combined with 1–2 tablespoons shredded cheese. In a snack bowl, spoon warm chili (such as Amy's Organic Canned Vegetarian Chili). Sprinkle with cheese and repeat process.

6. Very Berry smoothie*

7. Divide a snack bowl: Greek yogurt, whole grain cereal, diced fruit (fresh or canned in water/juice)

8. Divide a snack bowl: cottage cheese, a dash of cinnamon, whole grain cereal, diced fruit (fresh or canned in water/juice)

9. Half a graham cracker rectangle, spread thinly with nut butter or ricotta cheese, along with ¼ cup unsweetened applesauce.

10. Divide a snack bowl: frozen yogurt (or frozen yogurt drops) with six melon balls

11. Slice a melon in half. Use a melon baller to scoop watermelon, cantaloupe, or honeydew balls. Refrigerate leftover melon for 3–4 days.

12. Whole grain cereal with cow milk or unsweetened vanilla almond milk

13. Very Hungry Fruit Caterpillar: ¼ cup diced kiwi, one thin strawberry slice, three banana slivers, four chopped blueberries. Place strawberry head on plate. Arrange the diced kiwi in a wavy pattern to form a caterpillar body, attach blueberries as eyes and legs (you can use Greek yogurt for sticking), and bananas as a mouth and antennae.

14. Combine ½ chopped boiled egg with 2 tablespoons mashed avocado

15. Flax-Coated Fruit Dippers* with ½ serving of string cheese

16. Baked Cinnamon Apple* with a dollop of yogurt

17. Sweet Potato with Apple Sauce*

18. Cheesy grain with veggies: Divide snack bowl: steamed peas and carrots (from frozen package), cooked whole wheat macaroni or brown rice. Sprinkle 1–2 tablespoons shredded cheese over the top and microwave in 10 second intervals, until cheese is melted. Serve warm.

19. Veggie Slurpy: Warm up ¼ cup reduced-sodium canned soup made with pureed vegetables, such as carrots, butternut squash, tomato, or sweet potato. Let soup cool and pour into a sippy cup. Try healthy soups made by Imagine, Trader Joe's, Amy's, or Pacific.

20. Creamy Rice Pudding*

21. Red-White-Blue Cheese Bagel: Puree ½ cup fresh or frozen (thawed) mixed berries. Stir blended fruit with 8 ounces of reduced-fat cream cheese or part-skim ricotta cheese. Spread 2 tablespoons of cheese on mini–whole grain bagel. Makes four snack servings. Refrigerate leftover cream cheese in sealed container for up to five days. Use as a dip for bite-size banana or apple slices.

Roasted Veggie Chips

Active time: **10 minutes**
Cook time: **30 minutes**
Serves: 8

2 cups mixed vegetables, chopped (carrots, zucchini, yellow
    squash, broccoli florets)
1 tablespoon flavored olive oil (such as lemon, basil, or
    rosemary)
¼ -½ cup whole-wheat Panko breadcrumbs*
Hummus or marinara sauce (for dipping)
*Low in sodium and a good source of fiber, try 100% whole-
    wheat *Kikkoman Panko Japanese Style Bread Crumbs* for
    satisfying crunchy chips.

➤ Preheat oven to 425°F and coat a baking dish with cooking spray. In
a mixing bowl, toss the vegetables with olive oil until evenly coated.
Arrange vegetables in baking dish and sprinkle with breadcrumbs.
Bake 25–30 minutes, until vegetables are tender. Serve with hummus
or marinara sauce for dipping.

Very Berry Smoothie

Active time: **5 minutes**
Cook time: **None**
Serves: 4 (½ **cup servings**)

1¼ cups low-fat chocolate milk*
1½ cups frozen mixed raspberries, strawberries, blueberries
* For toddlers under 2 years old, use whole milk

➤ Place all ingredients in blender, cover, and whip until smooth.

Flax-Coated Fruit Dippers

Active time: **5 minutes**
Cook time: **None**
Serves: **2**

½ cup sliced fruit such as banana, pear, apple, or melon
Yogurt, for dipping
2 tablespoons ground flaxseed meal

➤ Dip fruit slices in yogurt. Place ground flax in a shallow baking dish
and roll fruit slices in dish until covered with coating.

Baked Cinnamon Apple

Active time: **5 minutes**
Cook time: **45 minutes**
Serves: **4**

1 medium apple
Pinch of cinnamon, for sprinkling

➤ Preheat oven to 400°F. Rinse apple, and with a small knife, slice the base so that the fruit can easily stand up. Using a paring knife, core the middle in a circular motion. Discard the inner seeds. Place apple on a baking dish with a few tablespoons of water on the bottom and lightly sprinkle with cinnamon. Bake for 45 minutes, until apple is "oozing" and easily pierces with fork.

Remove and let cool. Skin will peel right off. With a spoon, or ice scream scoop, divide apple evenly into four portions.

Baked fruit is a nutritious way to offer your toddlers a sweet ending to a meal. Leftovers can be mashed into breakfast cereal. Pears also work well in this recipe.

Sweet Potato with Applesauce

Active time: 5 minutes
Cook time: 8 minutes
Serves: 4–6

1 sweet potato
½ cup unsweetened applesauce

➤ Using a fork, prick holes on all sides of potato, and place in a microwave-safe bowl with plastic wrap. Poke a small hole in the wrap leaving an air vent. Cook on high for 8 minutes, turning halfway through cooking time. Slice open and let cool. Scoop out potato flesh. Combine with applesauce.

Creamy Rice Pudding

Active time: **5 minutes**
Cook time: **20 minutes**
Serves: **8 (¼ cup servings)**

2 cups cooked instant brown or white rice (90-second Uncle
    Ben's Ready Rice)
1½ cups 1 percent milk*
⅓ cup sugar
½ teaspoon ground cinnamon
Pinch salt
Mashed banana (optional topping):
*For toddlers under 2 years old, use whole milk dairy.

➤ Combine cooked rice, milk, sugar, cinnamon, and salt in medium
saucepan and bring to boil. Lower heat to simmer. Cook, stirring
occasionally until milk is absorbed, about 20 minutes.

    Transfer to a serving bowl and cool completely. Divide rice
pudding into eight portions. Stir in 2 tablespoons mashed banana if
desired.

PRESCHOOLER MEAL PLAN (AGES 3–5 YEARS)

What is the appropriate diet for your preschooler? In truth, it is no different from the diet we outlined earlier for your toddler. The American Academy of Pediatrics and the American Heart Association recommend that all children, thin, medium, or obese, be placed on the so-called "prudent" diet starting at age 2. This is a diet that is low in saturated fat and cholesterol and high in fruits, vegetables, and whole grains, with less fatty red meats and more lean meats, fish, and low-fat milk.

One problem with supplying your child with this nutritious, heart-healthy obesity prevention diet is that it is not available for many low-income families due to its cost. It is estimated that over 13 million low income Americans currently live in what are called "food deserts:" urban neighborhoods and rural towns without easy access to fresh, healthy foods. Instead of supermarkets and grocery stores, many of these communities are served only by convenience stores and fast-food restaurants that unfortunately offer very few nutritious foods options. The National Center for Health Statistics reported that young children in areas like this consume over 10 percent of their total calories in fast-food establishments. Of interest is that there was no difference with this caloric intake across socioeconomic classes.

Further complicating matters is the fact that energy dense junk foods are much less expensive than the lower energy nutritious foods that we recommend. One analysis showed that the cost of 1,000 calories for the energy-dense "junk" foods was a $1.76 compared to $18.60 for 1,000 calories of low-energy nutritious foods. Despite this cost difference, we strongly recommend that you make a strong effort to feed your young child the right way. The health difference will far exceed the extra dollars you spend.

The following are specific meal plans and snacks that will guarantee proper nutrition, help develop healthy eating habits, and work to protect your little child from becoming overweight or obese. Some of the principles that were discussed earlier will be repeated for emphasis, since they are very important.

The following menu, including meals and snacks, is designed for healthy preschoolers without dietary restrictions and is based on an average of 1,200–1,400 calories per day. Offer two to three daily snacks, especially for active preschoolers, spaced at least two hours apart from mealtime. Serve milk or water with meals and snacks. Two-and-half cups of milk (or dairy equivalents) every day will provide most of the calcium your preschooler needs for bone growth and still not interfere with an appetite for other foods. Serve skim milk, low-fat milk (1 percent), soymilk, or calcium-fortified unsweetened non-dairy milk.

WEEKLY MENU

Sunday

BREAKFAST

Quick Quinoa and Veggie Roll-Up

LUNCH

Yummy Tummy Soba Noodles
¼ cup edamame

DINNER

Buttermilk "Fried" Chicken and Waffles
½ cup watermelon cubes

Monday

BREAKFAST

Mini Crostini

LUNCH

Whole Wheat Couscous Cake
Zucchini Coins or Spaghetti Squash Lasagna

DINNER

Cheddar Chili
Whole Grain Mini Muffin

Tuesday

BREAKFAST

Swiss Egg-in-a-Hole

LUNCH

Cheddar Pear Grilled Cheese
Vegetable Matchsticks

DINNER

Chicken and Shrimp Tapas
Tomato-Glaze and Sweet-Ginger Glaze
Quick and Snappy String Beans

Wednesday

BREAKFAST

Multigrain Super Cereal

LUNCH

Salmon and Brown Rice "Sushi"

DINNER

Apple Chicken Quesadilla
Low-fat yogurt (½ cup)

Thursday

BREAKFAST

Quick Oats with Popped Amaranth

LUNCH

Waffle Falafel Bites
Hummus Veggie Piñata

DINNER

Quick Chicken Fiesta

Friday

BREAKFAST

Whole Grain Antioxidant Pancakes

LUNCH

Sweet and Savory Tacos
Avocado Herbed Egg Salad Tacos
Strawberry Lettuce Tacos

DINNER

Rainbow Spaghetti and Meatballs

Saturday

BREAKFAST

Choco-Butter Wake Up Smoothie

LUNCH

Incredible Hulk Pesto Pizza

DINNER

Oat Crusted Coconut Chicken Strips
Sweet Potato Fries

Quick Quinoa and Veggie Roll-Ups

Active time: **10 minutes**
Cook time: **15 minutes**
Serves: **4**

1 cup of uncooked quinoa
2 cups water or unsalted vegetable broth
12-ounce bag frozen blend: carrots, broccoli, cauliflower
4 (6-inch) whole grain tortillas
4 tablespoons flavored hummus or tomato sauce

➤ Add 1 cup of quinoa to 2 cups of broth or water. Bring to boil and simmer for 12–15 minutes, until liquid is absorbed. Set aside 1 cup of cooked quinoa in a bowl and refrigerate the rest for 3–5 days.

While quinoa is cooking, steam vegetables in microwave according to package directions. Let cool and chop vegetables into bite-size portions. Add 1 cup of vegetables into bowl with quinoa and stir together.

Microwave tortillas between two damp paper towels for 30–45 seconds each. Spread one tablespoon of hummus or tomato sauce on each tortilla and top with ¼ cup of quinoa-vegetable mixture. Starting at one end, roll-up the tortilla until tightly sealed. Cut into bite-size pieces and serve as a finger food.

This recipe yields about 2 cups each of leftover quinoa and vegetables, which can be used as hearty additions to canned tomato soup or as a topping on whole grain pizza crust.

Known as the "mother of all grains," quinoa has been a South American staple for centuries. Naturally high in protein, quinoa is technically an edible seed with impressive amounts of iron, magnesium, phosphorous, and folic acid. Before cooking, use a fine mesh strainer to rinse the quinoa and remove the outer coating, called saponin, which can give the quinoa a bitter taste. Mix quinoa with beans for a tasty side dish, or with stir-fries.

Mini Crostinis

Active time: **5 minutes**
Cook time: **2 minutes**
Serves: **1**

2 whole grain crispbreads* or 3 gluten-free rice cakes (corn, quinoa, brown rice)
Choose a topping: *(Choose reduced-fat cheese and yogurt)*
2 tablespoons ricotta cheese + ¼ cup mixed diced berries
2 tablespoons cottage cheese + ¼ cup diced pineapple (canned in water or juice)
2 tablespoons Greek yogurt + ¼ cup diced tomatoes and cucumbers
2 tablespoons goat cheese + 1–2 diced figs, dried or fresh
2 tablespoons crumbled feta cheese + ¼ cup diced watermelon
1 tablespoon almond or peanut butter + ¼ mashed ripe banana
1 slice Swiss cheese + ¼ cup chopped broccoli or asparagus cuts, frozen package
* Whole grain crispbreads and rice cakes are sold at local grocery stores and are available online—Wasa: www.wasa.com, Ryvita: www.ryvita.com, Suzie's Thin Cakes: www.amazon.com

➤ Let your preschooler help you decorate the crostinis! Choose a topping (look at the ingredients you have on hand) and spread evenly over crackers or rice cakes. If using frozen vegetables, steam in microwave according to package instructions. For preschoolers who prefer softer textures, you can use a mini–whole grain pita pocket stuffed with a "surprise" filling.

Crostini or "little toasts" are traditionally thin slices of baguette brushed with butter and baked. In this recipe, we use a hearty crispbread or rice cake as a canvas for a flavorful topping.

Swiss Egg-in-a-Hole

Active time: **5 minutes**
Cook time: **5 minutes**
Serves: **2**

1 tablespoon margarine made with vegetable oil
2 slices whole grain bread
2 large eggs
2 thin slices reduced-fat Swiss cheese, cut into circles

➤ Punch out a circle in the center of each slice of bread using a round cookie cutter or the bottom of a small drinking glass (save bread holes for snack).

Melt margarine in nonstick skillet over medium-high heat. Place two slices of bread in skillet. Crack an egg into each hole in the bread and cook until bottom sides are golden brown and egg firms up, about 2–3 minutes. Using a thin spatula, gently flip bread and cook the second side until egg is set about 1–2 minutes (keep the spatula against the skillet to release any stuck egg before turning over). Lower heat and melt each egg-in-a-hole with slice of cheese. Remove skillet from heat and serve.

> *Preschoolers can dig the egg out of the hole with a mini fork or use their fingers to break off pieces of bread and scoop it in the egg. Select margarines that are made from canola or olive oil, without "partially hydrogenated oil" on the ingredient list*

Multigrain Super Cereal

Active time: **5 minutes**
Cook time: **20 minutes**
Serves: 6

1 cup of mixed whole grains such as millet, teff, and buckwheat*
3 cups water
Cinnamon stick (optional)
1 cup warm soy, almond, 1 percent or skim milk, divided
1 cup chopped citrus fruit salad: strawberries, oranges, kiwi,
    divided

➤ In a medium saucepan, bring grains and water to a boil. Add cinnamon stick, cover and simmer on low heat until grains are tender and liquid is absorbed, about 20 minutes. Discard cinnamon stick.

Divide cereal between individual bowls and stir in ¼ cup warm milk. Serve with ¼ cup fruit salad. Leftover grains keep 3–4 days in your fridge and take minutes to warm up with just a little water. Toss a handful of cooked whole grains into soups, tacos, or whole grain wraps for an instant nutrient boost.

* When mixing grains, select whole grains with similar cooking times, such as quinoa and bulgur, using 2 cups of liquid. Blending whole grains delivers a unique nutrient package of protein, vitamins, minerals, and antioxidants—and pairing them with citrus fruit increases iron absorption. For a quick breakfast, pre-soak whole grains in water overnight to cut down cooking time.
You can purchase whole grains at your local grocery or health food store, or order online at www.grainplacefoods.com, *or* http://www.bobsredmill.com.
*   Millet resembles cornmeal in taste and is a light yellow-colored grain with a soft, fluffy texture- a good source of fiber, B-vitamins, magnesium, and phosphorus.*
*   Buckwheat is high in protein and has impressive amounts of magnesium, copper, and manganese. Buckwheat groats, which are hulled seeds from a plant related to rhubarb, are called "kasha."*
*   Teff comes as tiny red, white, or brown grains with twice the iron and three times the calcium of other grains.*

Whole Grain Antioxidant Pancakes

Active time: **5 minutes**
Cook time: **20 minutes**
Serves: **6–10***

¾ –1 cup whole grain pancake mix
* Depending on brand

Antioxidant Topping (per pancake)
1 teaspoon almond butter
¼ cup mixed berries with mashed ripe bananas
1 tablespoon Greek yogurt mixed with 1 teaspoon ground nuts,
    chia seeds, or flaxseeds

➤ Prepare whole grain pancakes according to package directions. Top each pancake with individual toppings.

Who needs syrup when you can top your pancakes with a sweet dose of health-boosting antioxidants? Whole grain pancake mix provides a shortcut to a healthy breakfast on busy mornings. You can find whole grain pancake mix at your local grocery store, natural food store, or order online at http://www.hodgsonmill. com, http://www.bobsredmill.com, or www.grainberry.com.

Choco-Nutty Wake-Up Smoothie

Active time: **5 minutes**
Cook time: **None**
Serves: **2 (1 cup servings)**

2 tablespoons 100 percent pure cocoa powder (Nestlé)
2 tablespoons creamy natural peanut butter (Hampton Farms)
1 medium, fresh, ripe banana
8-ounces nonfat vanilla Greek yogurt (Chobani®)
Dash of cinnamon
4–6 ice cubes

➤ Place all ingredients in blender, cover, and whip until smooth.

Quick Oats with Popped Amaranth

Active time: **1 minute**
Cook time: **1 minute**
Serves: **4**

1¾ cups 1 percent or skim milk, or Unsweetened Almond,
    Cashew, or Flax Milk*
1 cup Quick 1-minute Oats
Dash of cinnamon or nutmeg
1 cup mixed berries, fresh or thawed from frozen package

➤ Boil milk and add oats. Cook 1 minute over medium heat, stirring
occasionally. Sprinkle with cinnamon or nutmeg.
    While oatmeal cools slightly, prepare popped amaranth.

*Cow and Soy milk typically have 7–8 gram of protein per cup
and at least 30 percent of a day's calcium, 25 percent of a day's
vitamin D, and 20 percent of a day's vitamin B12. If your preschooler has a soy or cow milk allergy, alternative non-dairy milks
can serve as a healthy choice. Non-dairy unsweetened milk from
almond, rice, cashew, flax, hemp, and oat are lower in protein
(average 1–2 grams protein per cup), but select brands have added
calcium, vitamin D, vitamin B12, and are low in added sugar with
half the calories of cow milk—making them flavorful additions to
a balanced breakfast.

Try: *Silk Unsweetened Almond Milk—Original or Vanilla; Blue
Diamond Almond Breeze— Unsweetened Original, Vanilla,
or Chocolate; Trader Joe's Unsweetened Almond Milk—
Original or Vanilla; Silk Unsweetened Cashew Milk; Cashew
Dream Unsweetened Original; Good Karma Flax Protein
Plus Unsweetened, Original, or Vanilla Milk; Silk Almond
Coconut Blend Unsweetened Milk*

Based on nutrient values from *Nutrition Action Health letter January/
February 2015*

Popped Amaranth

Active time: **2 minutes**
Cook time: **10–15 seconds**
Serves: **4**

1 pot with lid
1 tablespoon amaranth seeds* (yields about 3 tablespoons
    popped)
* You can find amaranth at natural food stores or available
    online: www.bobsredmill.com, www.arrowheadmills.com or
    www.amazon.com

➤ Preheat pot over medium-high heat. Add a drop of water to pot; if
it "sizzles" you are ready to pop. Stir in amaranth and quickly cover
as amaranth starts to pop. Slide the pot back and forth just above
the burner. Uncover after 10–15 seconds and remove from pan. The
popped grains will look like tiny white beads. Sprinkle 1–2 teaspoons
of amaranth over oatmeal.

    Make more to store. Popped amaranth makes a crunchy yogurt
topping or can be added to a vegetable stir-fry seasoned with dried
herbs and grated parmesan cheese. When popping a larger batch,
always stir in amaranth **1 tablespoon at a time** (to prevent burning),
and follow the process described above.

*Amaranth is a tiny seed with super grain qualities—it's gluten-free
and contains all nine essential amino acids, making it a complete
protein. Amaranth is also a star source of iron, magnesium, and
phosphorous.*

*   Oats, a familiar whole grain, are a nutritional powerhouse of
fiber available as rolled, whole, steel-cut, or quick-cooking. Oats
boast polyphenol compounds that have antioxidant properties
and are a good source of protein and fiber.*

Yummy Tummy Soba Noodles with Edamame

Active time: **5 minutes**
Cook time: **10 minutes**
Serves: **4**

Soba Noodles
1 bunch of greens such as chard, spinach, collard, or kale*
4 cups reduced-sodium chicken or vegetable broth
2 cloves minced garlic, fresh or jarred
1 tablespoon extra-virgin olive oil
2 teaspoons of reduced-sodium soy sauce.
4 ounces dry soba noodles (half of an 8-ounce package, such as
    Eden Foods

Edamame
1 cup whole or shelled edamame (soybeans in pods) or ½ cup
    shelled, from frozen package

➤ Prep your greens: Rinse greens well. Cut or tear away the leaves from the stem. Coarsely chop. (Tip: Slice a bunch of greens in half lengthwise, discard stems and ribs. Roll leaves crosswise into a cigar shape. Cut crosswise into very thin slices with a sharp knife).

Heat a large skillet over medium heat and sauté garlic in oil for 1 minute. Add greens, tossing to coat, and cook until leaves are tender, 5–10 minutes, depending on your preference (spinach wilts quickly, in just 2 minutes). Stir in soy sauce.

In a large pot, bring broth to a boil, reduce to a simmer, and add the noodles. Cook until the noodles are tender, 5–6 minutes. Strain the noodles through a colander, reserving the liquid broth.

Divide noodles between small bowls. Break noodles into smaller strands if desired. Scoop ¼ cup chopped greens over noodles, ladle broth over mixture, and serve warm.

Steam edamame according to package directions. Serve whole edamame on the side or if using shelled edamame, chop and stir into the noodles with broth.

Also known as buckwheat noodles, soba noodles are a whole grain Japanese pasta served warm or cold. Edamame is an excellent source of plant protein, and your preschooler will love popping these steamed soybeans out of their pods. Whole edamame is safe for children with enough teeth to chew crunchy foods, but it should be cut into small pieces for younger toddlers to help prevent choking.

*Make more to store. In the South a large quantity of greens to serve a family is commonly referred to as a mess o' greens. Fresh-cooked greens can be refrigerated in airtight container for 3–5 days. Reheat and toss in chopped raisins and crushed pine nuts for a flavorful side dish.

Whole Wheat Couscous Cakes

Active time: **15 minutes**
Cook time: **15 minutes**
Serves: **10**

¾ cup cooked whole-wheat couscous, prepared from package
    and cooled*
2 cups canned pumpkin puree (not pumpkin pie filling)
1 egg
¾ cup whole grain cornmeal (Bob's Red Mill or Arrowhead
    Mills)
Dash of spice: cinnamon or nutmeg
¼ cup extra-virgin olive oil + cooking spray as needed
Plain Greek yogurt, for dipping
*1 cup dry couscous makes about 3 cups cooked. Refrigerate
    leftover couscous for 3–4 days.

➤ Prepare couscous according to package directions and place ¾ cup
in a mixing bowl. Stir in pumpkin, egg, cornmeal, and spice to form
batter. Heat olive oil in a nonstick skillet. Scoop ¼ cup portions of
batter and place in skillet, lightly flattening with a spatula. Cook 4–5
minutes per side.

Tip: Flip cakes over when edges start to rise. Add additional
cooking spray as needed. Serve with a dollop of yogurt.

*This recipe adds a creative twist to a classic pancake. Couscous
resembles a small, grain-shaped pasta. Whole wheat couscous can
usually be "cooked" simply by soaking in boiling water. You can
also use whole wheat farro (an ancient wheat popular in Italy,
Greece, and Rome) in this recipe.*

Crunchy Zucchini Coins

Active time: **10 minutes**
Cook time: **30 minutes**
Serves: **4**

1 medium zucchini
Cooking spray
Skim milk for dipping
2 tablespoons of grated parmesan cheese
¼ cup cornflake crumbs

➤ Preheat oven to 425°F. Wash zucchini. Slice into circular coins. Spray cookie sheet with cooking spray. Pour milk in one bowl and stir together parmesan cheese and cornflake crumbs in another bowl. Dip zucchini coins in milk and then coat with cheese and corn flake crumb mixture. Bake for 30 minutes, flipping halfway through cooking time. As a quick alternative, you can slice zucchini into thin matchsticks or coins and sauté with a few tablespoons of tomato sauce on the stovetop in a nonstick frying pan.

These sweet cheesy coins make an ideal light vegetable side dish or snack. Double the recipe and store leftovers for up to two days in the refrigerator. Summer squash peaks in summer and late fall. Varieties include zucchini, yellow (straightneck and crookneck) and pattypan and can be interchanged in most recipes.

Cheddar Pear Grilled Cheese with Vegetable Matchsticks

Active time: **10 minutes**
Cook time: **5 minutes**
Serves: **1**

2 slices whole grain bread
½ teaspoon extra-virgin olive oil
1 teaspoon all fruit preserves, any flavor
1 slice cheddar cheese
¼ pear, thinly sliced
½ cup mixed vegetables, sliced into matchsticks (carrots, cucumber, peppers)
1–2 tablespoons packaged hummus

> Brush one side of each slice of bread lightly with olive oil. Turn the bread over and spread one slice with fruit preserves; top with cheese and pear, then add remaining bread slice, oiled side up.

Lightly coat a griddle or large skillet with cooking spray. Preheat over medium heat. Add sandwich and cook for 5 minutes, or until cheese is melted, turning once to brown both sides. Cut into squares and serve with vegetable matchsticks and hummus.

You can transform your grilled cheese sandwich into fun shapes by using assorted cookie cutters. Try hearts, flowers, or favorite childhood characters such as Elmo and Mickey Mouse.

Salmon and Brown Rice "Sushi"

Active time: **10 minutes**
Cook time: **20 minutes**
Serves: **2**

Cooking spray
4 ounces salmon
¼ cup calcium-fortified orange juice
1 tablespoon + 1 teaspoon rice vinegar
2 teaspoons reduced-sodium soy sauce
1 teaspoon sugar
1 cup cooked brown rice *(Try 90-second Uncle Ben's Ready Rice or Boil in a Bag)*

➤ Preheat oven to 425°F. Place fish in a dish coated with cooking spray. Pour in the orange juice. Bake for 15–20 minutes or until fish flakes easily with a fork.

While salmon is cooking, in a small saucepan, bring the vinegar, soy sauce, and sugar to a boil. Remove from the heat. Stir in the cooked rice and let cool to room temperature. Flake the cooked fish with a fork into fine pieces and add to rice. Spoon half the rice mixture into a ½-cup measuring cup, packed tightly. Let your preschooler help you invert the molded rice salads onto a plate (similar to making sandcastles). Repeat process. Serve with a spoon or as a wrap.

> *Sushi rolls are tricky to make, but you can enjoy similar flavors in this kid-friendly recipe that features a simple baked salmon and brown rice mold. Your preschooler may also enjoy wrapping the rice mixture in whole grain tortilla strips or lettuce wraps as a mock sushi roll.*
>
> *You can substitute the salmon with 1 cup (about 8 ounces) firm tofu, patted dry with a paper towel, sliced into cubes. Sauté tofu on stovetop with 1 teaspoon canola oil and orange juice; combine with brown rice.*
>
> *It's always healthier for your toddler to eat their fruit rather than drink it—in this case orange juice is used to flavor-boost the salmon without adding excessive sugar.*

Waffle Falafel Bites

Active time: **15 minutes**
Cook time: **20 minutes**
Serves: **4**

Cooking spray
4 falafel patties, prepared from a falafel mix
1 tablespoon extra-virgin olive oil
2 omega-3 fortified eggs
2 tablespoons 1 percent or skim milk*
8 frozen mini whole grain waffles or 2 regular waffles, quartered.
4 tablespoons nonfat plain yogurt, divided*
* For 1–2 years olds, use whole milk dairy.

➤ Preheat oven to 400°F. Spray 2 baking sheets with cooking spray. Combine half a box of falafel mix with cold water as instructed on package. Form about 12 ½-inch thin patties and place on baking sheet. Lightly brush them with oil and bake for 8–10 minutes. Flip them over and bake 8–10 minutes longer, until browned. Set four falafel patties aside and refrigerate or freeze the rest.

While falafel is baking, whisk eggs and milk together in a bowl. Heat a nonstick skillet with cooking spray and scramble eggs over medium heat until fluffy. Divide egg mixture into four portions.

Toast waffles according to package instructions. Make a waffle sandwich by placing one mini waffle or waffle quarter on a plate. Top with falafel patty, ¼ egg mixture, and complete sandwich with other mini waffle or waffle quarter. For tiny hands, use a pizza slicer to make bite-size triangles. Alternatively, serve a "deconstructed sandwich" with individual components scattered on a plate. Let your preschooler have fun with this dish. Serve with yogurt as a dipping sauce.

Who needs bread when you can bite into a crispy waffle? This Mediterranean inspired recipe combines chickpea-based falafel balls with whole grain waffles and an egg in the middle for a high protein kid-friendly sandwich.

Suggested brands:
> *Falafel mix: Casbah, Fantastic Foods mix, or Veggie Patch premade falafel balls.*
> *Frozen Waffles: Earth's Best whole grain mini waffles, Van's 8 whole grain waffles*

Hummus Veggie Piñata

Active time: 5 minutes
Cook time: None
Serves: 4

1 bell pepper
½ cup each: sliced cucumbers and baby carrots
½ cup packaged hummus, any flavor

➤ Slice pepper in half, and scoop out inner core with seeds. Fill one hollowed out pepper slice with cucumber-carrot mixture and the other pepper with hummus. Press both peppers together to create a closed piñata and let your preschooler break it open. Tear the pepper into edible strips for dipping. Chop up leftover peppers and use in an egg omelet, grain pilaf, or a quick stir-fry.

This piñata is a great side dish for a group. For a single serving, use ¼ cup sliced vegetables and 1–2 tablespoons of hummus.

Avocado Herbed Egg Salad Tacos

Active time: **5 minutes**
Cook time: **12 minutes**
Serves: **1**

1 omega-3 fortified egg
¼ cup light mayonnaise made with vegetable oil
1 tablespoon chopped herbs: chives or basil
1 teaspoon minced garlic
1 (6-inch) whole grain tortilla
2 tablespoons ripe avocado, mashed
1 tablespoon reduced fat shredded cheddar cheese

➤ To hard-boil the egg, put the egg into a saucepan, and then add enough cold water to cover egg by ½ inch. Bring water to a boil over high heat. Remove from burner and cover pan. Let eggs stand in hot water, about 12 minutes. Run cold water into pot to stop cooking. Gently peel egg.

In a small bowl, combine mayonnaise with herbs and garlic. In a separate bowl, mash egg and stir in 2 teaspoons of the prepared mayonnaise. Spread tortilla with avocado and spoon egg salad mixture down the center. Sprinkle with cheese and fold taco in half. Wrap leftover avocado tightly in plastic wrap, sprinkle exposed flesh with a little lemon or lime juice to prevent discoloration, and refrigerate for up to 3 days.

Make more to store: Boil a batch of eggs, and refrigerate them shell-on for up to 1 week. Refrigerate leftover mayonnaise in airtight container for up to 1 week and use to flavor-boost chicken or tuna salads.

Strawberry Lettuce Taco

Active time: **5 minutes**
Cook time: **None**
Serves: **1**

½ cup fresh strawberries, chopped
1 teaspoon balsamic vinegar
¼ teaspoon ground black pepper
Pinch of black pepper
Fresh lime juice (from a small wedge, ¼ of a lime)
2 romaine lettuce "taco" leaves
1 tablespoon reduced-fat shredded mozzarella cheeses

➤ Stir together the chopped strawberries, balsamic vinegar, pepper, and lime juice. Divide mixture between lettuce wraps and sprinkle with cheese.

Incredible Hulk Pesto Pizza

Active time: 5 minutes
Cook time: 5 minutes
Serves: 1

1 tablespoon of tomato sauce + extra for dipping
1 ½ cups chopped spinach-arugula, from packaged salad blend
1 whole grain English Muffin
1 ½ teaspoons store-bought pesto
¼ cup reduced-fat shredded mozzarella cheese, divided
½ cup cauliflower and broccoli florets, from frozen packages
1 teaspoon grated parmesan cheese

➤ Preheat broiler. In a nonstick frying pan, warm up the sauce over medium heat. Sauté spinach and arugula until wilted, 2–3 minutes. Split a whole grain English muffin and brush with pesto. Spread spinach-arugula mixture evenly over each half and sprinkle with cheese. Broil until the cheese melts.

Steam vegetables in microwave according to package instruction. Sprinkle with parmesan cheese and serve with tomato sauce for dipping. Slice each pizza into four squares.

If you have time, here's how to make a batch of home-made pesto:
Makes: ¾ cup

2 tablespoons chopped pine nuts	4 cups basil leaves
2 garlic cloves, peeled	½ cup grated Parmesan-Romano cheese
3 tablespoons extra-virgin olive oil	¼ teaspoon salt
	Mini food processor

➤ With food processor on, mince the pine nuts and garlic. Add the remaining ingredients and blend until smooth.

You can refrigerate leftover pesto in an airtight container for up to 5 days. Alternatively, you can freeze single portions of pesto in ice cube trays or mini plastic snack bags for up to 3 months.

Spaghetti Squash Lasagna

Active time: **20 minutes**
Cook time: **15 (+20–80) minutes**
Serves: **9–12**
Roasted Spaghetti Squash is easy to prepare in the microwave or oven but plan on an additional 20-80 minutes of cooking time respectively.

Roasted Spaghetti Squash:
1 whole spaghetti squash

Lasagna:
4 cups roasted spaghetti squash
3 cups fresh or frozen chopped baby spinach
1 cup baby carrots (about 12) or 1 cup frozen
1 cup tomato sauce, divided
1 cup reduced-fat shredded mozzarella cheese, divided*
1 tablespoon grated parmesan (optional)

➤ *Roasted Spaghetti Squash*
Preheat oven to 375°F. Rinse squash and poke holes around the entire surface using a fork. Place squash on a foil lined sheet and bake in oven, turning halfway through cooking time. Remove and let cool.

Slice squash in half lengthwise. With a spoon, scoop out the inner seeds and discard. Using a fork, scrape out four cups "spaghetti" squash strands. Refrigerate unused spaghetti squash for three days or freeze for future use.

*Quick microwave method: Pierce squash all over with a small sharp knife. Place in a microwave-safe bowl covered with a damp paper towel; cook on high for 5 minutes, turn the squash, and repeat process 2–3 times until squash is tender, approximately 20 minutes (when a knife slides in pretty easily, the squash is done). Let cool. Slice squash in half lengthwise, scoop out inner seeds, and remove spaghetti strands.

➤ *Lasagna*

After roasting the spaghetti squash, preheat oven to 375°F. Cook frozen vegetables according to package instructions. If using fresh spinach, place in a microwave-safe dish, loosely covered, and cook for 3 minutes until leaves are wilted. Let cool slightly, chop spinach leaves, and set aside. Squeeze cooked spinach in paper towels to remove excess water. Steam carrots with 2 tablespoons of water in microwave-safe dish, loosely covered for 3 minutes. Mash with fork.

Prepare the Lasagna: Coat bottom of baking dish with a few tablespoons of sauce. Add a layer of spaghetti squash strands, ¼ cup of each vegetable, and ¼ cup cheese. Repeat process with sauce, squash, vegetables and cheese until you have four layers. Sprinkle top layer with parmesan cheese.

Bake uncovered until lasagna starts to bubble, about 15 minutes. Let cool and slice into lasagna squares.

Preschoolers make wonderful kitchen helpers—they can help spread, spoon, and sprinkle the lasagna ingredients! Make more to store—you can freeze half a batch of lasagna squares and nuke them for an instant meal on days when you need a healthy meal shortcut.

Buttermilk "Fried" Chicken Fingers and Waffles

Active time: **10 minutes**
Cook time: **30 minutes**
Serves: **8**

Cooking spray
1 cup low-fat buttermilk
1 cup whole wheat bread crumbs
¼ cup grated parmesan cheese
1 pound boneless, skinless chicken breasts or tenderloins, sliced
    into 8 strips
4 frozen whole grain waffles
Optional topping (per waffle): 1 tablespoon mashed bananas,
    berries, or applesauce

➤ Preheat oven to 400°F. Coat a roasting pan with cooking spray. Add a few tablespoons of water or low sodium broth on the bottom of pan to keep chicken moist throughout baking.

Pour buttermilk into a large bowl. In a separate bowl, mix breadcrumbs and cheese. Dip chicken strips in buttermilk and coat with breadcrumb mixture. Transfer chicken strips to roasting pan and arrange in single layer. Bake 10–15 minutes per side, until golden brown and cooked through.

Prepare waffle according to package directions. Cut waffles into quarters, for a total of 16 waffle bites. Top waffle bites with fruit topping. Serve with chicken strips.

Preschoolers will dive into this dish for a finger-licking crispy meal. Oven-frying makes this dish super healthy. You can marinate the chicken strips in buttermilk a day earlier and refrigerate in a sealed plastic bag overnight.

Cheddar Chili with Whole Grain Corn Muffins

Active time: **30 minutes**
Cook time: **20 minutes**
Serves: 8
This recipe is a kid-friendly version of classic chili with a little less of the spicy stuff, but filled with flavor from beans, herbs, and tomatoes. Use leftovers for a quick chili-cheese toast snack.

Corn muffins:
Whole grain corn muffin mix*
Cooking spray
Mini muffin tin
* Use a whole grain corn muffin mix, available at natural food stores: www.bobsredmill.com or ready-to-eat golden corn Vitatops: www.vitalicious.com

Chili:
1 pound 90 percent lean ground turkey or beef
2 tablespoons olive oil
1 onion, diced
2 minced garlic cloves, fresh or from jar
1 (14.5 ounce) can diced tomatoes in Italian herbs, undrained
1 (8-ounce) can tomato sauce
1 (15-ounce) can cannellini beans, drained and rinsed
1 (15-ounce) can red kidney beans, drained and rinsed

Toppings (per serving):
1 tablespoon reduced-fat shredded cheddar cheese
1 tablespoon reduced-fat plain yogurt

➤ Lightly grease a mini–muffin tin with cooking spray. Prepare corn muffins according to package directions. Let cool and set aside.
    In a chili pot, preheat olive oil over medium heat for 1 minute. Add the turkey or beef and cook for 5–6 minutes, using a spoon to

break up any large clumps of meat. Add the onions and garlic and sauté for 3–4 minutes. Stir in the tomatoes, tomato sauce, and beans. Reduce the heat to medium-low, cover the pot and simmer the chili for 20 more minutes. Ladle 1 cup of chili in a small bowl. Garnish with topping. Serve with corn muffin.

Shortcut: Use pre-cooked shredded rotisserie chicken (about 3 cups) instead of ground turkey.

For a savory touch: Add a ½ teaspoon of cinnamon or allspice to chili

Quick Chili Cheese Toast: Take a piece of whole grain toast, add a dollop of chili, and sprinkle with reduced-fat cheese. Broil for one minute.

Chicken and Shrimp Tapas

Active time: **10 minutes**
Cook time: **5 minutes**
Serves: **4**

Tomato-Glazed Tacos
1 cup broccoli florets, from frozen package
1 tablespoon olive oil
2 tablespoons tomato paste
2 tablespoons red wine vinegar
2 minced garlic cloves, fresh or from jar
½ teaspoon dried oregano
½ teaspoon dried basil
8 ounces boneless, skinless chicken breasts or shrimp, tail-off,
    peeled, and deveined
Cooking spray

➤ Prepare broccoli according to package directions. Let cool and coarsely chop.

In a bowl, combine the olive oil, tomato paste, red wine vinegar, garlic, oregano and basil. Cut the chicken or shrimp into 1-inch pieces and toss to coat in marinade.

Spray nonstick skillet or wok with cooking spray. Add chicken or shrimp and stir-fry for 4–5 minutes over medium heat until cooked through. (Cooked shrimp will turn opaque and chicken will no longer be pink). Stir in chopped broccoli.

Tapas are snacks, canapés, or finger food that originated in Spain and are served throughout the Mediterranean. As your preschooler grows into an independent eater, now is the time to introduce new flavor combinations and tapas are fun for the whole family to nibble on.
Tapas pairing, choose one:
Serves: 4

12 whole grain crackers with ¼ cup hummus
1 cup cooked bulgur or whole wheat penne, divided

Sweet-Ginger Glaze

Serves: 4

2 teaspoons peanut oil
½ teaspoon grated ginger, fresh or from jar
8 ounces boneless, skinless chicken breasts or shrimp, tail-off,
    peeled, and deveined
1 cup leafy greens, such as spinach or baby bok choy, sliced
2 tablespoons fresh lime juice
1 tablespoon reduced-sodium soy sauce
1 teaspoon honey

➤ Heat oil in nonstick skillet or wok over medium heat. Add ginger and cook 1 minute. Add chicken or shrimp and stir-fry for 4–5 minutes over medium heat until cooked through (cooked shrimp will turn opaque and chicken will no longer be pink). Stir in chopped greens and cook until wilted. Stir in lime juice, soy sauce, and honey.

Tapas pairing, choose one:
Serves: 4

4 (6-inch) whole grain tortillas
1 cup cooked brown rice, divided

➤ Spoon the filling down center of a warm tortilla, and fold in half or serve over rice.

Time savers: Use pre-cooked protein such as frozen shrimp (thaw and dice) or shredded rotisserie chicken and heat in microwave with marinade. Stock your pantry with jars of pre-minced garlic and ginger, which serve as instant flavor boosters.

Quick and Snappy Steamed Green Beans

Active time: **15 minutes**
Cook time: **10 minutes**
Serves: **4**

2 cups fresh or frozen chopped green beans
Water (for steaming)
1 teaspoon olive oil
1 tablespoon slivered almonds
½ cup sliced diced canned mandarin oranges + 1 tablespoon of
    liquid from can

➤ If using frozen green beans, steam in microwave according to package directions. If using fresh green beans, rinse and snap off stem ends with your fingers. Cut the green beans into uniform bite-size pieces. Add 1 inch of water to a saucepan and insert a steamer basket. The water should reach the bottom of the basket without touching it. Bring water to a boil and carefully arrange green beans in basket. Cover and steam over medium heat for 3–7 minutes, until tender.

In a skillet, sauté almonds in olive oil for 1–2 minutes until golden brown. Add the steamed beans, and stir in diced oranges with juice.

Green beans make an easy finger food snack served raw or simply steamed.

Apple Chicken Quesadilla

Active time: **10 minutes**
Cook time: **10 minutes**
Serves: **2**

1 apple
Cooking spray or 2 tablespoons of water
2 precooked chicken sausage links (85 grams each)
1 tablespoon extra-virgin olive oil
2 (6-inch) whole grain tortillas
2 slices of Havarti or Cheddar cheese

➤ Rinse the apple and slice into wedges, discarding the inner core with seeds. You can also use an apple corer for easy slicing. Lightly coat the bottom of a glass baking dish with cooking spray or water. Spread the apples in an even layer in the baking dish. Cover with plastic wrap and microwave for 3½–4 minutes. If apple slices pierce with a fork, they are done. If they don't feel soft, cook for an additional 30–60 seconds. Remove the plastic wrap, drain any water in the dish. Cut apples into bite-size pieces or mash it with a fork.

Slice sausage links into circles, and then cut into small bits. Heat a nonstick skillet with olive oil. Add sliced sausage and cook until heated through, about 5-7 minutes. Stir in cooked apples.

Microwave tortillas between two damp paper towels for 30 seconds. Spoon and spread apple-sausage mixture evenly on one tortilla. Top with cheese and second tortilla. Slice into four triangles.

Havarti is a versatile cow milk cheese that pairs well with fruit and works well sliced, grilled, or melted into dishes.

Select reduced-sodium cooked chicken sausage links, such as Al Fresco brand. Preschoolers are more likely to enjoy the milder, less spicy flavors such as sweet apple, roasted pepper and asiago, or spinach and feta.

Quick Chicken Fiesta

Active time: **15 minutes**
Cook time: **10 minutes**
Serves: **4**

12-ounce bag small baby white or yellow potatoes (about 12–13 potatoes)
1 (14.5-ounce) can diced canned tomatoes
6 ounces skinless cooked rotisserie chicken breast, shredded into bite-size pieces
1 cup shelled edamame, from frozen package
1 tablespoon tomato paste
½ cup reduced-fat shredded mozzarella cheese

➤ Remove the potatoes from the package and pierce them with a fork. Place them in a microwave-safe bowl with plastic wrap and then poke a small hole in the wrap. Microwave on high for 5–6 minutes or until fork tender. Cooking time may vary slightly depending on your oven. Slice potatoes into bite-size pieces. Cook edamame according to package directions.

Heat a large nonstick skillet over medium-high heat. Add diced tomatoes, chicken, and edamame and heat 1–2 minutes. Stir in potatoes and tomato paste and cook additional 1–2 minutes. Stir in cheese until melted through.

Rainbow Spaghetti with Meatballs

Active time: **30 minutes**
Cook time: **20 minutes**
Serves: 8

Zucchini Spaghetti:
1 green zucchini
1 yellow zucchini
Handheld spiralizer
1 tablespoon extra-virgin olive oil
1 tablespoon grated parmesan cheese
2 tablespoons of vegetable broth or tomato sauce (if making puree)

Meatballs:
1 tablespoon extra-virgin olive oil
1 pound 90 percent lean ground beef
½ cup part-skim ricotta cheese
1 egg
¼ cup whole wheat bread crumbs
1 tablespoon fresh or 1 teaspoon dry dill, chopped
2 cups tomato sauce

➤ Insert green zucchini into spiralizer and twist (like a pencil sharpener) into spaghetti strands. Repeat process with yellow zucchini. Break spaghetti into smaller strands, if desired. Toss vegetable strands with olive oil and cheese. Place mixture in microwave-safe bowl with plastic wrap and then poke a small hole in the wrap. Cook for 1 minute, stir and cook for additional 30 seconds until softened.

Preheat oven to 450°F. Drizzle olive oil in a baking dish to coat surface. In a large bowl stir the beef, ricotta, egg, breadcrumbs, and dill to create a meatball mixture. Roll the mixture into eight round balls and line them up in rows on baking sheet. Bake for 20 minutes until the meatballs are cooked through. Heat tomato sauce in saucepan and pour over cooked meatballs. Slice meatballs into bite-size pieces or mash with fork and serve with rainbow spaghetti.

A spiralizer is one of my essential kitchen gadgets that easily converts vegetables into spaghetti strands. Any raw vegetable such as carrots, squash, or cucumbers can be used to instantly create fun-to-eat veggie spaghetti. You can purchase the Premium Slicer Spiralizer for under $15.00 on Amazon.

Crispy Coconut Chicken Fingers

Active time: 15 minutes
Cook time: 30 minutes
Serves: 4

Cooking spray
½ cup oats or ground flaxseed meal
½ cup grated parmesan cheese
¼ cup unsweetened coconut flakes
1 large egg
8 ounces boneless, skinless chicken breasts, cut into strips
Drizzle of honey (optional)

➤ Preheat oven to 400°F and coat a baking sheet with cooking spray. If using oats, place oats in a food processor and process for 20 seconds, until coarsely ground. In a mixing bowl, combine ground oats or flaxseed meal with cheese and coconut flakes.

Beat egg. Dip chicken strips in egg and dredge in oat or flaxseed mixture. Arrange chicken fingers on baking sheet in a single layer, lightly drizzle with honey and cook 10–15 minutes per side, until golden brown.

Sweet Potato Fries

Active time: **10 minutes**
Cook time: **25 minutes**
Serves: **4**

1 sweet potato
Cooking spray
2 teaspoons extra-virgin olive oil
Pinch of salt, pepper, cinnamon

➤ Preheat oven to 425°F. Scrub potato under running water and with a vegetable peeler remove tough areas of skin, leaving most of the skin intact. Slice potato into ¼–½ inch sticks. Arrange potatoes in a single layer on baking sheet coated with cooking spray. Lightly brush potato slices with olive oil and sprinkle with seasoning. Bake for 25 minutes, turning halfway through cooking time, until potatoes easily pierce with a fork.

A healthy snack portion is based on a 4-ounce bowl or plastic food container, unless otherwise specified. Snacks marked with an * are accompanied with a recipe. For dairy snacks, select reduced-fat yogurt and cheeses, skim, 1 percent; soy; or unsweetened non-dairy milks.

1. Divide a snack bowl into mini whole grain crackers, Easy Guacamole* (or packaged), bell pepper strips

2. Bunless BLT*

3. Cheese Broomstick* or Cheese Flag* with ½ cup milk

4. Black bean taco (Serves 2): Spread a thin layer of plain yogurt or mild salsa on a 6-inch whole grain tortilla. Top with ¼ cup black beans, two thin slices of avocado, and 2 tablespoons of shredded cheese. Fold and broil until cheese is melted. Slice into triangles.

5. Protein in a Pita: Scramble an egg with two chopped grape tomatoes in cooking spray. Sprinkle with 1 tablespoon shredded mozzarella cheese. Scoop into a mini whole grain pita.

6. Melon Sailboat in the Sea: ¼ cup blueberry yogurt, five blueberries, one unsalted pretzel stick, one small melon wedge (sliced into a triangle), one orange wedge. In a snack bowl, add yogurt and top with blueberries. Poke the pretzel stick through the melon wedge to create a "sail". Insert the sail into the orange wedge to complete the sailboat and place on top of a blueberry sea.

7. Fruit Salad Pizza*

8. Black-Eyed Peas, Salsa, and Chips*

9. Quick Chili Cheese Toast: Top one slice of whole grain toast with 1–2 tablespoons of chili (refer to chili recipe or try Amy's Organic Canned Vegetarian Chili). Sprinkle with 1 tablespoon shredded cheese. Broil for one minute.

10. Fancy Canned Soup: Heat up ½ cup canned reduced-sodium soup made with pureed vegetables: carrots, butternut squash, tomato, or sweet potato. Stir in 2–3 tablespoons of cooked whole grains, chopped baby spinach or steamed peas and carrots. Try healthy soup brands such as Imagine, Trader Joe's, Amy's, or Pacific.

11. Divide a snack bowl: mini whole grain crackers, sliced cucumbers, Roasted Red Pepper Spread* or 1 tablespoon packaged hummus

12. String cheese, 1–2 tablespoons packaged bean dip or fruit flavored salsa, bell pepper or carrot sticks

13. Elvis Peanut Butter Toast: Spread one slice whole grain toast with ½ tablespoon peanut butter and ⅓ mashed ripe banana. Alternatively, you can use sesame seed, almond, or soy nut butter.

14. Choco-Nutty Wake-Up Smoothie*

15. Sweet Potato Fries with a cheese stick

16. Baby Eggplant Chips* with ½ cup milk

17. Wonton Chips* or one graham cracker rectangle with dip: ½ cup unsweetened applesauce or 1 tablespoon packaged hummus.

18. Banana Bits* or Banana Nut Butter Pop: Slide two unsalted pretzel sticks into two banana slices. Spread the top of each banana slice with 1 teaspoon of nut butter and stick on oat cereal. Serve with ½ cup milk.

19. Heart Sandwich Minis: Using a heart-shaped cookie cutter, punch a heart into one slice of reduced-sodium ham or turkey and one slice of reduced-fat cheese. Arrange thin slices of apples, strawberries, or pears on each heart and seal together to make a sandwich.

20. Oat Fudge Almond Drops* with ½ cup milk or yogurt

Easy Guacamole

Active time: **10 minutes**
Cook time: **None**
Serves: **8 (makes about 1 cup)**

1 ripe avocado
2 tablespoons each: finely chopped white onion, plum tomato
1 tablespoon chopped cilantro
1 garlic clove, minced (optional)
Pinch of salt
Fresh lime juice, to taste

➤ Slice avocado in half, discard inner pit; scoop out the flesh with a spoon. In a mixing bowl, mash avocado with a fork and add other ingredients, mixing well. Let the mixture stand for a few minutes before serving to allow the flavors to blend. Serve 2 tablespoons as a snack with whole grain crackers and vegetables.

Bunless BLT

Active time: **3 minutes**
Cook time: **3 minutes**
Serves: **1**

1 slice nitrite-free turkey or veggie bacon (such as *Morningstar
   Farm* or *Applegate Farms*)
1 tablespoon shredded lettuce
1 tablespoon diced tomatoes
1 slice reduced-fat cheddar or provolone cheese

➤ Prepare bacon according to package instructions, and crumble it.
Sprinkle bacon, lettuce, and tomato on cheese slice and roll it up.
Alternatively, use a lettuce wrap and fill with cheese and other
ingredients.

NUTRITIOUS NIBBLES FOR PRESCHOOLERS

Cheese Broomstick

Active time: **2 minutes**
Cook time: **None**
Serves: **1**

1 reduced-fat cheese stick
3 unsalted pretzel sticks
1–2 tablespoons marinara sauce, for dipping

➤ Cut cheese stick into thirds to create three "brooms." Insert pretzel stick by poking a hole in on one end of each cheese broom. Peel down the other end of the cheese into strands to create "broom strings." Let your preschooler "sweep" each broom in the marinara sauce.

Cheese Flag

Active time: **2 minutes**
Cook time: **None**
Serves: 1

1 round cheese, such as *Babybel*
2 unsalted pretzel sticks

➤ Slice cheese in half to create two semicircles. Poke a hole in each cheese wedge with a pretzel stick to create a flag.

NUTRITIOUS NIBBLES FOR PRESCHOOLERS

Fruit Salad Pizza

Active time: **5 minutes**
Cook time: **2 minutes**
Serves: **2**

1 whole grain pita, 6-inch tortilla, or flatbread
2–3 baby spinach leaves, torn into bite-size pieces
½ cup chopped strawberries or watermelon
2–3 tablespoons crumbled feta or goat cheese
Drizzle of balsamic vinegar (optional)

➤ Assemble pizza: Spread the spinach and fruit evenly over bread or tortilla. Sprinkle with cheese. Drizzle with vinegar. Broil until cheese melts. Slice pizza into four triangles.

Black-Eyed Peas, Salsa, and Chips

Active time: **5 minutes**
Cook time: **15 seconds**
Serves: **4**

½ cup canned black eyed peas, drained and rinsed (or white
    beans)
½ cup canned diced tomatoes
¼ cup reduced-fat cheddar cheese
2 ounces of whole grain tortilla chips* (about 10 chips per
    ounce, depending on brand)
1 cup vegetable sticks (carrots, bell peppers)
* Look for whole grains as the first ingredient on the food label,
    including chips made from whole wheat, whole corn, brown
    rice, quinoa, or spelt.

➤ Combine peas with tomatoes in a microwave-safe bowl. Top with
shredded cheese and cover bowl loosely with plastic wrap. Microwave on high for 10–15 seconds until cheese is melted. Serve with
chips or vegetable sticks.

*In the South, black-eyed peas are traditionally eaten as the first
food of the New Year to bring good luck and prosperity.*

NUTRITIOUS NIBBLES FOR PRESCHOOLERS

Roasted Red Pepper Spread

Active time: **5 minutes**
Cook time: **None**
Serves: 8

8-ounce package reduced-fat cream cheese or part-skim ricotta
    cheese
8-ounce jar roasted red peppers, drained
¼ cup grated parmesan cheese

➤ Using a mini food processor or handheld immersion blender, pulse
ingredients until smooth.

Choco-Nutty Wake-Up Smoothie

Active time: **5 minutes**
Cook time: **None**
Serves: 4 (½ cup servings)

2 tablespoons 100 percent pure cocoa powder (Nestlé)
2 tablespoons creamy natural peanut butter (Hampton Farms)
1 medium, fresh, ripe banana
8-ounces nonfat vanilla Greek yogurt (Chobani®)
Dash of cinnamon
4–6 ice cubes

➤ Place all ingredients in blender, cover, and whip until smooth.

Baby Eggplant Chips

Active time: 10 minutes
Cook time: 30 minutes
Serves: 6–8

2 baby eggplants or 1 medium eggplant
Cooking spray
1–2 teaspoons flavored olive oil (basil or rosemary oil)
¼ cup whole wheat panko breadcrumbs, for sprinkling
Marinara sauce, for dipping

➤ Preheat oven to 425°F. Wash eggplants. Cut off ends and make thin slices for a total of 16 circles. Slice the circles in half for a total of 32 "half-moon" shapes. Spray cookie sheet with cooking spray. Arrange eggplant slices in single layer and drizzle with olive oil. Sprinkle with panko. Roast for 30 minutes until slightly browned.

Panko adds a satisfying crunch to this delicious after-school snack, while baby eggplants have a more delicate skin and flesh, making them a kid-friendly choice. If using a larger eggplant, some bitterness can be removed by slicing and sprinkling the cut slices with salt. After about 10 minutes, blot and gently rinse the eggplant well.

Wonton Chips

Active time: **10 minutes**
Cook time: **10 minutes**
Serves: **8**

Cooking spray
24 wonton wrappers
Vegetable oil, for light brushing
Mini cookie cutters such as hearts, teddy bears, or fun shapes
Seasoning: sesame seeds, ground flaxseed, cinnamon, or dill for
    sprinkling

➤ Preheat oven to 350°F. Spray baking sheet with cooking spray. Lightly
brush wonton wrappers with oil. Use cookie cutters to punch shapes
from each wonton wrapper for a total of 24 chips. Sprinkle chips with
assorted seasonings. Bake chips for 5–7 minutes, until golden brown
and crisp. For a snack, serve 3 chips with applesauce or hummus for
dipping.

Banana Bits

Active time: **5 minutes**
Cook time: **5 minutes**
Serves: **4**

Cooking spray
1 ripe banana
Pinch of cinnamon, for sprinkling
2 tablespoons of crushed nuts
4 tablespoons of reduced-fat ice cream, any flavor

➤ Preheat a grill pan with cooking spray. Peel banana and halve lengthwise. Sprinkle with cinnamon and with a spatula, gently transfer to grill plan. Grill until browned and cooked through, about 2 minutes on each side. Remove from heat and sprinkle with nuts. Cut banana into uniform bite-size pieces. Divide banana bits into four portions and dip into ice cream.

> *A classic banana split gets a makeover in this recipe that features fruit as the centerpiece, with just a dollop of ice cream for dipping.*

Oat Fudge Almond Drops

Active time: **20 minutes**
Cook time: **5 minutes**
Serves: **3 dozen (36 drops)**

3 cups uncooked oats, quick or old-fashioned
½ cup creamy almond butter
1 teaspoon vanilla extract
1 stick vegetable oil margarine (such as I Can't Believe It's Not
    Butter or *Earth Balance Vegan Buttery Sticks)*
2 cups sugar
½ cup cocoa powder
½ cup 1 percent milk

➤ Line two baking sheets with waxed paper. Combine oats, almond butter, and vanilla in a mixing bowl. Melt margarine in a saucepan over medium heat and add sugar, cocoa, and milk. Bring to a boil and cook, stirring continuously for 2 minutes. Remove from heat and pour over reserved oat mixture. Stir until ingredients are well blended. Drop batter by tablespoons onto baking sheets for 18 drops; let cool at room temperature. Once fudge drops are firm, slice or easily break in half, carefully removing from waxed paper to serve. Fudge drops will keep in fridge for up to 3 days in a sealed container.

Create a "baking station" with a mixing bowl, spoon, and assorted measuring cups, and help your preschooler pour and stir ingredients together.

Remember that snack foods should be nutritious extensions of a meal. Serve healthy snacks that consist of a blend of whole grains, proteins, fruits, and vegetables.

QUICK TIPS TO
LIGHTEN UP MEALS

MAINTAINING A HEALTHY WEIGHT DEPENDS on achieving energy balance. This is accomplished by balancing the amount of energy burned and food consumed throughout the day. If your child has a body mass index approaching the 85th percentile or above, *now* is the time to introduce small changes in the types of food eaten and encourage fun ways to be more physically active each day. By offering a variety of healthy options and encouraging portion control (using child-size sectioned plates) at meal and snack times, your child will achieve energy balance without formally "dieting." Classic childhood favorites such as pizza, peanut butter sandwiches, or spaghetti and meatballs can still be part of a healthy eating pattern (with a few minor ingredient swaps). You can also avoid the "short order" cook routine by slimming down one recipe for the entire family—without compromising taste or nutrition.

Here are some quick, easy changes you can make to your child's diet that will put them on the path to lifelong health:

1. Use a nonstick skillet and a spritz of cooking spray for sautéing or preparing eggs in place of butter or margarine.

2. Use skim milk or calcium-fortified non-dairy milk in smoothie recipes.

3. In casseroles that call for cheese and milk, use reduced-fat cheese, 1 percent or skim milk. If a recipes calls for 1 cup of cheese, use ½ cup instead.

4. Use nonfat or low-fat Greek yogurt in recipes that call for sour cream.

5. Offer fruit as a dessert (½ cup apple slices with low-fat vanilla yogurt) instead of high sugar cookies and ice cream.

6. Serve plant-based entrées on most days of the week. Zucchini spaghetti with tomato sauce or bite-size carrot coins and broccoli trees with melted, reduced-fat shredded cheese are appealing to children.

7. Limit recipes featuring starchy vegetables (such as corn and potatoes) to 2–3 times per week.

8. Use unsalted broth or tomato sauce instead of oil for stir-fry dishes and purees.

9. Use whole grains as a "condiment." For example, instead of serving pasta as an entrée, add a few tablespoons of whole wheat macaroni to a vegetable stir-fry or sprinkle brown rice into chicken lettuce tacos.

10. Prepare dishes using a variety of lean proteins such as seafood, beans, tofu, skinless poultry, and 90 percent lean ground beef and ground poultry.

11. In baked goods, use applesauce or prune puree for half of the called-for butter, shortening, or oil. You can also replace half the fat for other moist ingredients that complement the flavor of your recipes, such as low-fat Greek yogurt, fat-free sour cream, low-fat buttermilk, orange juice, low-fat Greek yogurt, and light cream cheese.

12. In baked goods, you can usually substitute whole wheat flour for half of the white flour. Compared with ¼ cup of white flour, each ¼ cup of whole wheat flour adds 3.5 grams of fiber.

13. In baked goods, you can cut the sugar by a quarter and the recipe will still work out. For each tablespoon of sugar you cut out, you save 48 calories.

14. In baked goods, you can replace half of the eggs called for in a recipe with egg substitute. For each large egg that you replace with ¼ cup of egg substitute, you shave off 45 calories. If eggs aren't the

main ingredient, other foods can work in place of an egg, such as ¼ cup applesauce, ½ banana, or a mixture of 1 tablespoon ground flaxseed mixed in 3 tablespoons of warm water.

15. Lighten up omelets, frittatas, or scrambled eggs by substituting half of the eggs called for with 2 egg whites or ¼ cup egg substitutes.

16. Bulk up on antioxidants and fiber in your dishes with pureed fruit and vegetables. Puree or shred broccoli and cauliflower and use for spaghetti sauces, meatloaf, casseroles, whole grain pizzas, and sandwiches. Puree apple, peaches, pears or berries and spoon over fish, poultry, pancakes, or yogurt. Top fish or poultry with fruit salsa made from mango and lime, pineapple and cilantro, or peach and basil.

17. Skim the fat off soups, stews, and sauces before serving.

18. Pick water-packed tuna instead of tuna packed in oil.

19. Select soft, 6-inch taco whole grain tortillas instead of the larger burrito size.

20. Grill portabella mushrooms as a main or side dish in place of meat, or use mushroom caps instead of pizza crust. Remember to cut it into bite-size pieces!

FINAL WORDS

WOULD LIKE TO END THIS book by discussing three important, recently published studies that further strengthen my approach to the problem of childhood obesity:

The first study, from Ohio State University, analyzed 8,550 preschoolers. Those who were exposed to eating evening meals together as a family, who got enough sleep, and who had limited television time, were found to have a significantly lower prevalence of obesity as compared to the children who were not exposed to those three household routines.

The second study, from the Netherlands and published in the medical journal *Childhood Obesity*, is a systematic review and meta-analysis of all the published studies to date meeting their criteria for inclusion. Out of 11,250 identified articles, only 27 were included. The analysis of these studies, involving over 1,000 overweight or obese young children, demonstrated that treatment programs targeting lifestyle changes in diet, physical activity, and behavioral modifications were most effective.

The third study, published in 2015 in the *Journal of Pediatrics*, involved a large group of 2–4 year olds and targeted four behaviors that lead to obesity: 1) milk consumption, 2) juice and sweetened beverage consumption, 3) TV/screen time, and 4) lack of physical activity. A follow-up after 12 months showed that in the targeted group, the half that were specifically counseled about these four behaviors showed a decreased rate in their BMI percentages as compared to those who were not targeted.

The point is that the early obesity prevention principles that I have discussed in this book are simple to carry out and they *work*. This is not nuclear physics or rocket science. Every parent is *more* than competent enough to follow my guidelines.

There is no question that the early prevention of obesity is both easier and more successful than waiting to treat older children who are already overweight or obese. During these early years, you as parents have more control over your child's daily environment. A large component of childhood obesity is established by the age of 5. The sooner your child learns to eat an appropriate, nutritious diet—low in high-calorie sugary foods and drinks—and develops vigorous physical activity habits, the greater her chances of never having to fight the difficult, often unsuccessful battle against obesity.

The ball is in your court. Game on!

THE 10 COMMANDMENTS FOR "WINNING THE OBESITY BATTLE"

1. Monitor your child's weight percentile regularly

2. Encourage outdoor physical activity each day

3. Less TV

4. More sleep

5. Cut down on juice

6. No soda or sweetened fruit drinks

7. Healthy snacks

8. Never use food as reward

9. Nutritious, well-balanced diet

10. Eat family meals together

APPENDIX

BMI Charts for Boys and Girls (Ages 2–20)

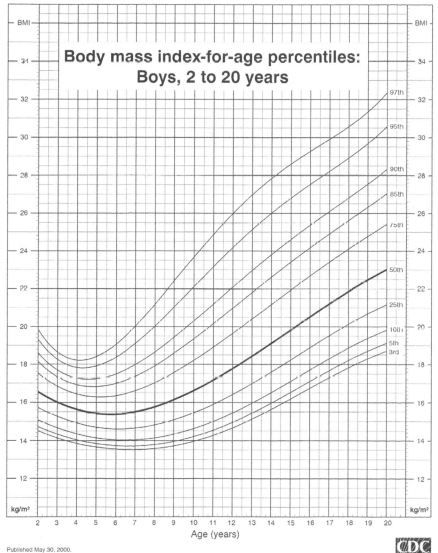

Body mass index-for-age percentiles: Boys, 2 to 20 years

Published May 30, 2000.
SOURCE: Developed by the National Center for Health Statistics in collaboration with
the National Center for Chronic Disease Prevention and Health Promotion (2000).

CDC
SAFER·HEALTHIER·PEOPLE™

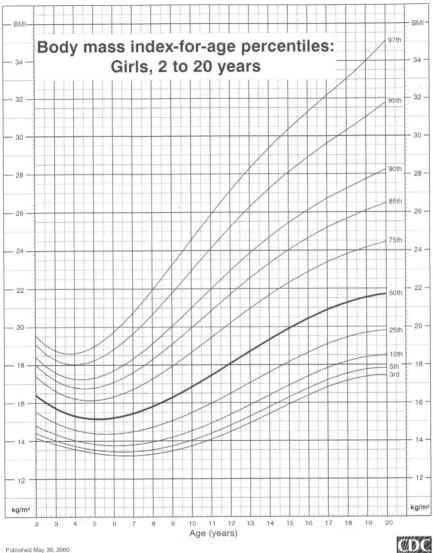

Body mass index-for-age percentiles: Girls, 2 to 20 years

Published May 30, 2000.
SOURCE: Developed by the National Center for Health Statistics in collaboration with
the National Center for Chronic Disease Prevention and Health Promotion (2000).

SAFER·HEALTHIER·PEOPLE™